Mind Myths

Awakening to a New Freedom from Chronic Illness and Emotional Distress

by Jeffery Scott Sullender, Ph.D., CCN

"There are three classes of people: those who see. Those who see when they are shown. Those who do not see."
Leonardo da Vinci

© 2012 Clinical Nutrition Press, LLC.

All rights reserved. No parts of this book may be used or reproduced by any means, graphic, electronic, or mechanical, including photocopying, recording, taping or by any information storage retrieval system without the written permission of the copyright holder.

Contents

Introduction v
What This Book Is and Is Not xvi

Part I – The Starting Point 1

Chapter 1 – Has Your Mind Been Captured? 2

Part II – The True You 7

Chapter 2 – Who Are You? 8
Chapter 3 – The Real You 12
Chapter 4 – Escaping from the Three M's 18
Chapter 5 – The Power of Symbols 23
Chapter 6 – Creating Opinion By Creating Crises 31

Part III – The Power of Perspective 35

Chapter 7 – Creating Our Perspective 36
Chapter 8 – An Act of Surrender 41
Chapter 9 – Recalibrating Our Perceptions 44
Chapter 10 – Sound Creates Form 51
Chapter 11 – A Rose by Any Other Name 54
Chapter 12 – Conscious or Subconscious? 60

Part IV – Identity and Belief 63

Chapter 13 – You and Your Health 64
Chapter 14 – Identity and Health 66
Chapter 15 – Placebo's Evil Twin 70
Chapter 16 – Revealing Our True Beliefs 72
Chapter 17 – The Name Game 76
Chapter 18 – Growth or Sour Grapes 78
Chapter 19 – When it Hurts to Change 80
Chapter 20 – A Few Words About "The System" 89
Chapter 21 – Believe It or Not 102
Chapter 22 – The Seven Self-Soothing Delusions 104

Part V – The Conceptual Myths in Health and Disease 115

Chapter 23 – Conceptual Myth #1: Normal or Common 116
Chapter 24 – Conceptual Myth #2:
        Genes Control Your Health 119
Chapter 25 – Conceptual Myth #3:
        The Illusion of Side Effects 123
Chapter 26 – Conceptual Myth #4:
        Modern Medicine or Good Medicine 127
Chapter 27 – Conceptual Myth #5:
        The Balanced Diet is All You Need 134
Chapter 28 – Conceptual Myth #6: Trust the Experts 140
Chapter 29 – Conceptual Myth #7:
        Public Health Policy Is the Best Policy 144
Chapter 30 – Conceptual Myth #8: False Evidence
        Appearing Real (F.E.A.R.) 156
Chapter 31 – Conceptual Myth #9:
        You Can Save Time and Money 161
Chapter 32 – Conceptual Myth #10:
        Modern Medicine IS Medicine 166
Chapter 33 – Conceptual Myth #11:
        Choice and the Law of Causality 171

Part VI – Personal Emancipation:
Reclaiming Your Power 177

Chapter 34 – Reclaiming Your Power 178
Chapter 35 – Challenge Your Current Health Paradigm 181
Chapter 36 – Expanding Your Personal Power 184
Chapter 37 – Daily Action Steps 202
Chapter 38 – Personal Action Steps 207

Part VII – Epilogue 211

Glossary 215

Appendix A 219
Appendix B 223

Introduction

People are changing. Without a doubt, there is a global awakening going on in almost every corner of the world. Little by little, people are beginning to emerge from their trance-like slumber to see a very different picture of their world. People are beginning to look behind the curtain of what they have been shown and see connections they had not seen before. We want to have control and authority over our lives, over our bodies and over our personal health. We want to eat and drink what we believe is best for us and to access those treatments that we have determined for ourselves to have merit. We are looking to invest in products that match our values. We want authenticity and integrity in our friends, in government and in society's institutions. We are highly sensitive to being misled or deceived. And as a result of this new vision, we are making changes in our lives and networking with others of like mind. An awakening is occurring among the peoples of the earth, and those who have held power have taken notice.

United States Presidential advisor Zbigniew Brzezinski, in his book *Between Two Ages: America's Role in the Technetronic Era,* speaks to the fact that for the first time in all of human history "almost all of mankind is politically awake, activated, political, conscious, and interactive". He goes on to say that while there were a "few pockets of humanity here or there in the remotest corners of the world" which were not yet politically awake, there was a "world wide search in the quest for personal dignity and cultural respect in a diversified world, sadly accustomed, for many centuries, to domination by one portion of the world of another". That observation is profound.

But as people awaken, many do so into a state of anger. They realize, perhaps for the first time in their lives, that they have been misled and that things are not as they appeared. They now realize that they cannot trust the banks or the bankers; they cannot trust the medical industry; they cannot trust their government; they cannot trust the giant transnational corporations that have taken control of their food and energy; and they cannot even trust that researchers and scientists have not sold their souls to the interests that sponsored them. In short, the people and institutions they relied upon have failed. A healthy, functioning society is based on a foundation of trust—earned trust, not blind trust. When that trust is betrayed, people end up hurt.

So many of our daily choices and actions are based on a highly complex system of unspoken beliefs about health, science, our bodies and the society we live in. This system of beliefs constitutes our personal map of the world—the world as we see it based on our experiences and what we have been told. Many of the beliefs that comprise our personal map are concepts, assumptions and attitudes that we have never given much active thought or even seriously questioned. Nevertheless, they function as the operating system and reference book we depend on throughout our lives.

In most cases, these beliefs are not even the product of our own design. They have been imprinted upon our minds through our interactions with significant people in our lives, such as parents, grandparents, teachers and religious figures. Our parents taught us what they knew based on their map of the world in order to help us become part of society; they wanted us to "get ahead" and "become successful." Society, meanwhile, wishes to imprint its rules, requirements and expectations on the minds of its members in order to foster some basic level of harmony. Of course, the media and television play a large role in this process. Whether those teachings are true or false or even beneficial to *you* is another matter. Later in life, a personal crisis arises to highlight the conflict between our experience of life and those rules and values society wishes us to follow. At that time, we begin to experience the need to examine both the source of our distress and the perceptions from which that distress arises.

Examining our own beliefs and assumptions tends to be curiously difficult. Most people will avoid it at all costs, even if doing so means continued suffering. We defend what we believe. We gather knowledge to make us feel safe, even if that knowledge is not always true. Even people who think of themselves as enlightened can have real difficulty when faced with truths that challenge their core beliefs. Often, the result is that they slip into a trance-like state of quiet acquiescence. As Sigmund Freud said, "Most people do not really want freedom, because freedom involves responsibility, and most people are frightened of responsibility." Years later, Sir Winston Churchill said, "Men occasionally stumble over the truth, but most of them pick themselves up and hurry off as if nothing ever happened." To challenge the beliefs and attitudes that we have been taught are true requires a degree of courage and personal honesty. The product of our personal examination will depend on our honesty and level of investigation.

The concepts and ideas that I present in this book represent a synthesis of my current understanding, experiences and perceptions that have arisen from my personal journey and from the tens of thousands of consultations I have conducted with clients over the last thirty-plus years practicing as a board-certified clinical nutritionist. Although I do not hold myself out to be a trained mental health counselor or psychologist, I have had an extraordinary opportunity to observe which attitudes and perspectives have served clients well and which have not. As in all human-to-human interactions, there is an exchange, and my clients and I share and learn from each other.

Many practitioners in so-called alternative or natural medicine find that a high percentage of their patients or clients are dealing with complex, multi-symptom, multi-system chronic illnesses. Many are essentially refugees from the conventional medical system. Some have been abandoned by conventional medicine as hopeless, untreatable, chronic, or non-compliant patients. Others have simply found that many of the treatments and drugs that were prescribed for them did nothing to address their real, underlying health issues and, in fact, frequently made matters worse.

So, what were the underlying issues? Broadly speaking, I found that after a couple of consultations I could place almost all of my clients into one of two categories: 1) those who needed additional information in order to experience improvements in their health, or 2) those who already had enough information, but were unable to move forward nonetheless. More simply stated, there were those who simply did not know and those who knew enough but still could not do anything.

In the early, pre-Internet years, I found that providing clients with additional information about what to eat, which supplements to take, etc., would make a tremendous difference. At that time, it was primarily a lack of knowledge and personally relevant information that held people captive in poor health. Later, access to information improved, and so-called Googling symptoms became more common. However, the additional information did not always translate into improvements in health. Providing those clients with even *more* information did not always help correct the underlying issue. Clearly, in these cases, an information deficit was not the problem. In fact, many were actually on information overload already. Another approach had to be developed. This new approach required a change in perspective. Information is only useful when interpreted in the appropriate context, and context is shaped by perspective. Throughout today's society, people and organizations are drowning in information. Yet this information is only useful when interpreted within the appropriate context.

Another more perplexing issue became apparent. Most clients professed an earnest desire to get well and insisted that they wanted to use natural methods to the greatest degree possible. However, a small number of these same clients would never do what was recommended. There were a number of reasons why they could not follow the program: they did not like vegetables, they did not have time in the morning to prepare a good breakfast, they got too busy at work to eat lunch, the "green drink" tasted too "green" and so on. For some of these clients, it was their first exposure to clinical nutrition as therapeutic modality and they simply did not know what to expect. Others may have expected to get well "naturally" by taking one or two "key" nutrients while continuing to consume their favorite processed foods, drinking just one less soda per day and maintaining the same lifestyle habits that degraded their health to begin with. In both examples, it was their underlying expectations that sabotaged their success. Success with clinical nutrition is predicated on two fundamentals: *knowing* followed by *doing*. From time to time, some clients get stuck in the "knowing" phase and just cannot progress to the "doing" phase. By gaining insight into our unspoken beliefs, we can avoid these frustrating outcomes.

My goal in writing this book is to offer help to the many people who feel stuck—those who have tried just about everything and are still ill in some way. I believe that by examining some of the beliefs and old programming that are operating in the background, these people may ultimately free themselves from the physical or emotional conditions that haunt them. There are dozens and dozens of nutrition and natural health books that can provide more so-called facts. This book is *not* one of them. Instead, this book focuses on my conviction that by changing our perspective, analyzing our subconscious beliefs and truly appreciating our vast personal power and potential, many more people can attain a vibrant and energetic level of health. Seeing things differently, through a totally different lens, can make all the difference in the world. As Einstein said, "No problem can be solved from the same level of consciousness that created it."

But altering our perspectives can be challenging, because we frequently bump into some of our core beliefs. So, a word of caution is necessary here to those readers who are strongly wedded to their preconceived concepts and beliefs, which may have their genesis in religious teachings, a public education, professional training or strong parental imprinting: This process can be uncomfortable, and you may have difficulty with some or all of the material presented in this book. I do not profess that what I say within this book represents some ultimate or exclusive truth. Nor would I presume to tell anyone what they should or should not believe. My goal is to pose the questions necessary to raise that which is beneath consciousness and bring it to consciousness. Although I have gone to great lengths to choose my words and symbols carefully, I cannot guarantee that the message intended will be the same as the message received. Thus, I must hope that these pages serve to point *toward* the truth as you can see and understand it. Take what serves you at this time; disregard the rest.

This book is divided into seven parts with Part II devoted to exploring the question of who *you* are. The need to focus on who you are is a critical step we all must take before we can understand our relationship to illness and disease. If you do not know *who* you are, how can you achieve any degree of freedom from an illness and all of the fears, beliefs and imperatives that often go hand in hand with being given a diagnosis? There is a vast difference between saying "I am depressed" and saying "I am having some feelings of being depressed."

Indeed, in the quest to achieve a greater degree of freedom in your life, including freedom from chronic disease, we must first start by freeing the mind. For it is within our mind that we have both accepted and assembled a vast network of assumptions that we regard as truth, but that often does more to enslave us than to free us. For a multitude of reasons, the bulk of the population has lived most of their lives in a trance-like state, conquered by Weapons of Mass Distraction—sports, entertainment, media, gossip and drama—and hypnotized by television programming and addictive technologies. For without our knowing or our conscious consent, our thoughts and perspective on life are being shaped by influential forces that many of us do not see and have not questioned. These forces directly affect how we think of our body, disease, health, healing and more.

As a result, many of us will spend the larger part of our lives sitting in a prison cell; because we cannot see the bars, we will have accepted the illusion that we are free. Our modern bias is to believe what we see and hear, especially if it comes from so-called experts. Also, we believe 100% in what we believe. When we view the world from the perspective of lack and limitation, we can only see those choices and options that fit into the perception of a limited reality and thus reinforce the very limitations that we wrestle against. To paraphrase Henry Ford, whether you believe you can or believe you can't, either way, you are right! This concept is nowhere more evident than in how we approach and understand health and disease.

My sincere hope is that the concepts and perspectives that I share in this book will help liberate readers from these personal prisons, whether that prison is experienced as a physical limitation, a medical diagnosis, the torment of chronic anxiety or depression or the belief that your life is small and you are powerless in the greater scheme of the Universe. I believe that you already know everything in this book on some level, even if only subconsciously. We are all born knowing, but have merely forgotten or were taught to forget. I also believe that every man and woman on this planet, no matter what country they are born into or in which culture they live, is endowed with unique gifts, talents, abilities, perceptions, insights and powers of creativity and that, with conscious intention or not, their mission in life is to uncover and develop these gifts for the benefit of all. To the extent that any human is bound by the slavery of chronic pain, illness, poverty or suffering, we all suffer, for we all lose the precious benefit of those gifts and contributions they would bring into the world.

True healing is an inherently holistic process. The idea that you can choose to heal one part of you and ignore another is fatally flawed and, over the long term, doomed to disappointment. Clients do this all the time. They want to work on their acne problem (because it shows) but do not mention their constipation and gas because they believe those issues are less important or even normal. Of course, you can selectively mask, cover or suppress symptoms via pharmaceutical or even natural means, but genuine healing involves all of you, mind and body, and it is a process, not an event. This concept is hardly new. The Greek philosopher Plato (429-347 BC) spoke of this when he said: "The cure of the part should not be attempted without treatment of the whole. No attempt should be made to cure the body without the soul. Let no one persuade you to cure the head until he has first given you his soul to be cured, for this is the great error of our day, that physicians first separate the soul from the body." True healing is intimately tied to our true potential: through health and the process of healing, a person is then free to access their full potential, and it is that potential that can change the world.

But what is health? How do we define "healthy"? In modern medicine, health is typically defined as the absence of disease, which oddly makes health a "negative state". In the real world, how many patients visit their physicians with a host of complaints, including fatigue, intestinal gas, hemorrhoids, recurrent headaches, dry skin and chronic anxiety? How many of these same patients undergo a battery of blood tests and even x-rays, only to be told that all the tests were "negative"? Often, the physician announces such results as, "Well, the tests say you are perfectly healthy!" But you went to the physician for a reason and this statement implies that the symptoms are imaginary or not real. But tests can only identify an abnormality, not the presence of health.

Therefore, the most honest answer a physician can offer is: "The tests that were ordered did not indicate the presence of any particular disease process at this time." Certainly, not every possible illness can be anticipated, so not every possible test would have been ordered. Further, as any biologist understands, physiology is not binary. That is, we do not move from a state of perfect health to having a disease in an on/off, yes/no manner. Twenty years before the diagnosis of Type II diabetes can be given, the patient moves ever so gradually through a progressive gray zone on their way to reaching the agreed-upon laboratory indicators required to award the new diagnostic label: diabetic! In fact, many patients who visit their physician while in that pre-disease or pre-pathology condition are effectively told to come back when things get worse!

The World Health Organization (WHO) defines health as follows: "Health is a state of complete physical, mental and social well-being and not merely the absence of disease or infirmity." That definition is an improvement over the concept that health is the absence of disease, but it still holds problems. In the July of 2011 issue of the *British Medical Journal,* Machteld Huber and colleagues illustrated this concern in saying: "Most criticism of the WHO definition concerns the absoluteness of the word 'complete' in relation to wellbeing. The first problem is that it unintentionally contributes to the medicalisation of society. The requirement for complete health would leave most of us unhealthy most of the time." True enough, but this argument goes even further. With the advent of on-demand full-body CT scans and high-resolution MRIs, we can now identify minor anatomical irregularities and other so-called defects that would never otherwise be known and might never lead to a specified disease. Nonetheless, these harmless variations are not considered normal.

So where do we draw the line? How do we include in our definition of health the immeasurable qualities of life that are not necessarily physical, such as peace of mind, self-confidence, a sense of purpose in life, a sense of identity, feeling loved, being able to give love, compassion and understanding? Are these qualities not important parts of wellness and health? Just because these attributes cannot be measured in a blood test or visualized through medical imaging technology, are we obligated to continue to discount them in our pursuit of optimal health?

All of us have the power to become healthy by virtue of being the magnificent creators of our lives. How can I make such a bold statement? Because it comes from my personal experience. In my late teens and early twenties, I experienced an escalating number of severe health problems that were becoming more disabling each month. Each tentative diagnosis was more distressing than the previous one. But as a pre-med major and a biologist, I was imbued with the conviction that science (as I knew it) and medicine would provide the answers. In my search for a cure, I consulted top specialists from several well-known teaching hospitals and clinics. I dutifully, if not enthusiastically, swallowed every new drug that was prescribed. Yet, with each consultation, procedure and new drug, my symptom picture only worsened. (Where was the placebo effect when I needed it?)

It was not until I endured another round of invasive tests and spoke with the top gastroenterologist at a major university hospital that I received my wake-up call. He said, "Well, Jeff, we really don't know what's going on with you. Either you will just get well or you will get sicker and die. We really won't know until the autopsy." That was quite a statement for a 22-year-old graduate school student to hear, and I think I was in a glassy-eyed fog for about week after that meeting. While this experience does not speak much to that physician's bedside manner, his words were *exactly* what I needed to hear and spoken *exactly* the way I needed to hear them. Had he been more sensitive and said something like, "Well, Jeff, I think there is a poor probability that you will fully realize your wellness potential… let's just wait and see," I do not think I would have gotten the message, and who knows if I would be writing these words today.

This encounter was the turning point in my path toward recovery and, as I came to realize much later, in my life. Somehow I was transformed from being a *follower* to a *seeker*. I was inspired and compelled to peek behind the curtain in medicine, healing and other facets of life. As a result, I suddenly found myself on what would turn out to be an eight-year journey to discover my own answers. That journey was certainly full of ups and downs and what I think of now as *cosmic irony*. As a biologist and with all the wisdom that a twenty-something could muster, I had been an outspoken critic of all things natural—homeopathy, herbal remedies, changes in diet and so on. I had ridiculed and rejected them all! After all, I was trained in science, which taught that these modalities were clearly bogus. Over those next eight years, as I took responsibility for my own health, my journey forced me to come face to face with each of the purportedly bogus treatment methods that I had previously eschewed. Ultimately, my healing came through everything I did not originally believe in! And so *Mind Myths* is not the product of some abstract academic pondering. Rather, *Mind Myths* emanates from my own personal journey of healing—a journey that continues to this day.

But first things first. The first step on this journey, your journey, is to realize your power and exercise it wisely.

What This Book *Is* and *Is Not*

I recognize that the concepts and content of this book will not resonate with everyone, which is usually the case with books that challenge accepted norms. *Mind Myths* was written and intended for those who are either curious enough or desperate enough to question what they see, what they have been taught, and why they remain where they are. *Mind Myths* is not intended to present an argument to change your mind. That job is entirely up to you. The footnotes common to academic writing have been omitted in deference to resource lists at the end of the book. The curious reader will be prompted to research those points that they question or feel challenged by. Meanwhile, the disengaged reader will simply read the words and go about their business, unchallenged and relatively unchanged. Those who approach this material through their predominantly intuitive nature should find the ideas most liberating and possibly inspiring. You will know on some level what makes sense to you. Those whose predominant perspective of the world is through a left-brain, logic-driven, or 3-D reality base are frequently the most challenged. The wild card is that you just never know when someone suddenly gets it. If that someone is you, then congratulations!

If I have done my job, something I present in the next pages will really get your dander up and challenge what you think or believe. As Gloria Steinem "The truth will set you free, but first it will piss you off". You may decide to modify what you believe, or you may decide to reject what I say. Either response is fine. I would not presume to tell you what you should believe, and nothing in these pages is intended to endorse or recommend any particular religion or spiritual belief system. What you believe is entirely up to you, and if you are growing and learning through your life experience, your beliefs and perspective will grow and change as well. I simply hope that you will examine such beliefs *consciously* and determine whether they serve or hinder you.

Mind Myths has no political agenda and is not intended as a political commentary or political argument. It is neither left nor right, neither conservative nor liberal. Yet whenever you discuss alternative medicine or complementary medicine, you are inevitably and probably unwillingly compelled to examine issues that have political overtones. Since the 1960s, it seems that just about everything has been politicized. I present this caveat at the beginning of the book to defuse some of the potential charge that political activist readers may hold.

Part I

The Starting Point

Chapter 1

Has Your Mind Been Captured?

How we see what we call "reality" may be less about the state of our physiology than the effects of our experiences and conditioning. The primary goal of this book is to help the reader see a more accurate picture of the reality that has been hidden and obscured. The unclouding of our vision will allow us to see the path to improved health, greater happiness, and our individual and collective freedom.

There is no definitive indicator to determine whether your mind, and hence your perception of reality, has been skewed or even captured by the messages you have been given. But there are indicators that can help provide insight. Ultimately, the ease or difficulty with which the reader can grasp and internalize the concepts and steps presented in this book will provide much of the evidence needed. The more difficulty the reader experiences, the greater the degree of programming that has occurred. That is neither an insult nor a slight against either one's character or intelligence. Consciousness has nothing to do with intelligence or academic degrees, nor is it tied to any geopolitical or cultural group. We are all awakening from our years and even generations of living in an orchestrated haze, and we are emerging at different speeds. Being "faster" or "slower" is of no importance. The fact that you *are* awakening and are willing to become more awake is what is paramount. When speaking of consciousness, it is important to define and differentiate what we mean. While the dictionary offers a definition of consciousness that is merely contrasted to a state of being unconscious, as might be the case with anesthesia, the quality of Consciousness of which I speak, denoted with a capital "C", is that quality of greater awareness and knowing resulting from a higher level of evolutionary development. Such a state is often developed in conjunction with certain virtues, such as patience, kindness, compassion, clarity, generosity, truthfulness, humility and forgiveness towards one's fellow man. Consciousness is, of course, a relative state and not a final destination.

Leonardo da Vinci once said, "There are three classes of people: those who see. Those who see when they are shown. Those who do not see." DaVinci was born on April 15, 1452 and is regarded as one of history's most ingenious inventors and creative thinkers. He was a painter, sculptor, architect, musician, scientist, mathematician, engineer, inventor, anatomist, geologist, cartographer, botanist and writer with a gift for genius. He conceptualized the helicopter, the military tank, parachutes, gliders and solar power. He stated that the Earth was not the center of the solar system (before Galileo Galilei was even born) and created numerous paintings and sculptures, including his famous *Last Supper*. He was the quintessential Renaissance man—and he never went to school. Consciousness and the process of awakening do not emanate from the limitations of the 3-D world or formal education.

Here are a few points that may provide evidence that you are awakening:

- You are increasingly frustrated that the only so-called healthcare you can obtain from the medical system is pharmaceutical or surgical, which you understand only addresses the symptoms of your condition and not the underlying cause;

- You find it increasingly unacceptable that the agencies that have taken on the role of protecting you are doing little more than protecting you from making your own decisions. The choices that you are not allowed to make may include your desire to drink farm-fresh raw milk, to identify and avoid genetically modified (GMO) foods, to treat your child's illness with nontoxic methods, to freely decline vaccinations, and so on;

- You find it increasingly difficult to find anything worth watching on television. Between the mind-numbing drivel that is presented as entertainment or the distorted nonsense that is presented as news, the television has become increasingly painful to watch or even listen to. You have learned that you can obtain what news you need from independent, uncensored sources, and there is better entertainment in a good book;

- You find it increasingly peculiar that you are forced to wear some sort of uniform to perform your work, such as a shirt and tie for men or some other specific dress code designed to impress co-workers, clients or customers;

- It strikes you as increasingly strange that each month, the media, in collaboration with Big Pharma, celebrates a particular disease or condition through a flurry of public service announcements and sponsored walk-a-thons purportedly to raise money for a cure. However, nobody wants to talk about where that money goes and what it actually funds, and there is never money raised to find the *cause*;

- You begin to find it increasingly illogical that parents should be intimidated, coerced and threatened into vaccinating their children when there are potentially serious consequences to any vaccination. And you cannot understand why some governments protect vaccine manufacturers by making them exempt from legal action when people are injured;

- You find it increasingly hypocritical that some so-called environmental experts who try to convince you that taking a hot bath or keeping your thermostat way up set to 66 degrees in winter is damaging the earth while at the same time they travel around the globe in fuel-guzzling private jets or caravans of SUVs and maintain multiple mansions that are comfortably heated and cooled year-round for their occasional enjoyment; or

- You find it increasingly incomprehensible that, at this point in human evolution, a sizable segment of humanity lives subordinated to the rule of certain individual men or women who, by sheer accident of birth, were born into a family that claims both a superior power and natural right to tell them how they will live and what portion of their labor they will contribute via taxes and fees. Queens? Kings? Princes? Royal Families? Really? In 2012?

The list could go on. But if any of these points resonate with you, then you are well on your way to greater Consciousness as a prelude to making a difference. When we speak of making a difference in the world, it is helpful to reflect on the phrase often attributed to Mahatma Gandhi: "Be the change that you wish to see in the world."

However, you may still be deep asleep if you believe:

- If it were not safe, it would not be for sale;

- Life expectancy in the US is increasing due to medical science;

- Medical science is working on a cure;

- You can safely rely on the experts, who will tell you what is best for you;

- Paying for a nice dinner out, your large HDTV, your motorcycle, your 108-channel cable television service and your convertible sports car is normal, but someone else should pay for your CT scan, your annual physical, your eye exam and your medications;

- Government intervention into healthcare will decrease costs and improve quality;

- Most serious illnesses are genetic, so you really cannot do much about them;

- You live in a free country; or

- You are free to make up your own mind.

Part II

The True You

Chapter 2

Who Are You?

The first step in the quest for freedom from disease begins with an understanding of *you*, including who you think you are and how you see yourself. This discussion is our first important and foundational step toward an understanding of symbols and identity and their relation to health and disease, as you will come to see.

If you ask most people the question "Who are you?", the most likely response you will receive is a declaration of their name: "I am Bill" or "I am Susan". Naturally, such an answer is entirely sufficient for social settings and the ordinary interactions of life. But such an answer conceals a greater question not answered in the response and which further prevents us from asking the question again in search of a deeper answer.

The asking of the question "Who are you?" is not merely an exercise in rhetoric or a fanciful journey in circular reasoning. It is, in fact, not only a fundamental question by which we define ourselves, but also the basis for our interaction with the world around us. Not knowing who we really are creates a powerful void within our Consciousness and leaves us vulnerable to the concepts created and promulgated by others. When accepted, such concepts contribute to the creation of a vast, invisible network of thoughts, beliefs, attitudes, values and expectations that do more to enslave us than free us. Achieving freedom in one's life, including freedom from chronic disease and disability, freedom from emotional suffering, freedom from poverty, freedom from manipulation and freedom of thought and expression, stems from our concept of self, meaning how we see ourselves as individual people and in relation to society, the world and the universe. As you will see, truly knowing who you are is difficult when you are constantly being told that you are someone else.

So, let's return to our opening question: "Who are you?" Although it may come as an initial surprise to you, you are not "Bill" or "Susan" or any other name you now use. Your parents gave you that name around the time of your birth, which is why it is called your given name, of course. Perhaps later in life you adopted a different name. Either way, you can answer to a name, but you cannot *be* a name. In this case, the Spanish language is more correct in asking, "¿Cómo se llama usted?", literally translated as "How do you call yourself." Furthermore, you can change your name whenever you wish or be known by more than one name at one time. At work you may use "William", as on your birth certificate, but your friends call you "Bill", and your brothers or sisters call you "Billy". You could also change your name to Harry or Margaret or Sky or Rain. And while it is relatively easy to change your name, did you change *you*? After all, a name is merely a social contrivance used to make a distinction between the Consciousness that is you and that of someone else. Your name is no more *you* than your jacket or your shirt.

So, when we ask, "Who are you?" for a second time, we may now try to answer by saying, "I am a man" or "I am a woman". Such answers may in fact be biologically correct, but in reality merely describe certain attributes of your physical body. But there is much more to you, isn't there? Let's try again. We may now offer up answers to the question with "I am a mother" or "I am a lawyer" or "I am an engineer" or "I am a husband". Yes, each of these answers may be totally true, but now we are attempting to define ourselves by the roles we currently play in our lives. Yes, perhaps at the current time, you may function in the role of "father" or "mother" to a child, or as "husband" to a wife and work in the role of "architect" or "engineer". But who were you before you assumed that role? You were *you*.

The desire to answer the question "Who are you?" could also prompt answers on yet another level, such as: "I am flesh and blood" or "I am energy" or "I am Spirit" or "I am Spirit having a physical experience" or any number of similar answers. True? Perhaps, but do you know this is absolutely true? Or is this answer just a strong belief or an assumption based on yet other beliefs?

You may also endeavor to define yourself by your beliefs: "I am a conservative" or "I am a socialist" or "I am a democrat" or "I am a Christian" or "I am a Buddhist". What does that really mean? Do you identify with those descriptions because that's how you were taught to identify yourself? Did you choose those beliefs on your own? What would happen if you asked ten different people: "What is a conservative?" or "What is a Christian?" How many different answers do you think you would receive? Would any of those answers agree with your understanding of the term? Would they even agree with each other? Would the answers to those very same questions be different if asked the questions 50 years ago to a different generation of people? The fact is that an identity based on a loosely defined and ever-changing label that is subject to great personal variations in interpretation can never be *who* you are. At best, such labels may approximate what you believe at the moment you answer, but in all reality your ideas about what you believe will evolve or change anyway. You may *have* a set of beliefs, but you cannot *be* a set of beliefs. So all you really know is that you exist and that you are conscious.

In early centuries, people identified themselves by the clan into which they were born. Clans or tribes may be ethnic, cultural, genetic or a combination of all three. In primitive times, knowing which tribe you belonged to, which tribes were friendly and which tribes were hostile was important knowledge for survival. People from other tribes were generally not trusted. They were outsiders or foreigners. People of like kind and like mind gathered together as the forerunners of today's nation-states. Mingling outside of the clan was limited and sometimes cause for being ostracized from your own clan. Even today, we still mistrust strangers as people from outside our clan. Nationalities are clans on a grander scale, and people try to identify themselves as "American" or "Japanese" or "German". Curiously, people tend to establish identity by defining differences, especially if there is pride attached to that identity. This tendency is often expressed in what we call nationalism or patriotism. Differentiating your beliefs from those of the tribe of clan is a longstanding source of conflict. Friedrich Nietzsche made this observation on this issue in stating: "The individual has always had to struggle to keep from being overwhelmed by the tribe. If you try it, you will be lonely often, and sometimes frightened. But no price is too high to pay for the privilege of owning yourself."

Today, we still tend to identify ourselves by the modern-day clan identities referred to as "nationalities". But what happens when you change your nationality? Do you change? Are you different because your world-defined clan membership changed? Certainly, the circumstances, opportunities and challenges that go with your new nationality will change, such as language, social norms, traditions, food and so forth, but did the essence of who you are substantially change? Probably not. As someone once said, "No matter where you go, there you are."

Chapter 3

The Real You

Did you ever say to yourself something like, "I really drive myself crazy" or "I can't stand myself"? Did you ever ask who is being driven crazy here? Who is the "I" in that thought that you can't stand? Doesn't such a statement imply there are two of you? Or, perhaps, two parts of you? Were you ever self-employed? Here again, there had to be two of you (an employer and an employee), since you cannot contract with yourself.

When we are actively thinking, we usually do so utilizing that voice we hear in our heads as we sift through information and make conscious decisions. We believe that the constantly chattering voice is who we are, when actually it is not. That voice in our head has been described in various terms, such as the ego, the left brain, the conscious analytical mind or the voice of knowledge. That voice loves to observe and examine details in a nearly endless stream of chatter, such as: "I'm hot. I hope the restaurant has air-conditioning. Look, the parking lot is nearly full. I wonder if they will have any lobster left? Maybe we should have called for a reservation? I'm hungry. I hope we can get seated quickly" and so on. If you are listening to that voice in your head, then who is doing the talking and who is doing the listening? And why would you have any need to tell yourself anything anyway? No, the real *you* rests in the silent Consciousness *behind* that voice, the place from which your thoughts and inspirations come forth even before your mind is aware of the thought.

Research in neurophysiology tells us that before we consciously make a decision, we have already made that decision at the subconscious level. So, how did that decision get made, and exactly who made it? How could it have been made before you consciously became aware of it?

Many of the sages of the ancient teachings say that the real you is found in the silence, in the momentary pauses between the long strings of nearly incessant thoughts that flow within our conscious mind. For this reason, many ancient spiritual and religious teachings emphasize the value of meditation or contemplative practices to quiet the mind and access that deep vault of riches and understanding that eludes the conscious linear mind. You cannot hear your intuition if your head and life are constantly full of outside distractions. You need quiet to hear that true voice of inner guidance, but you have to choose to hear it, and you have to practice hearing it. The external, manufactured world will do everything it can to entice you with 24/7 distraction.

One of the primary reasons why we may have difficulty developing a true understanding of who we are is that for most of our lives we have listened to people around us telling us that we were someone else. We have worn the mask of the actor in the many roles we play, and, in doing so, we have forgotten who is wearing the mask. The belief that you are only a body or a name becomes a self-made prison, and you become an unwitting slave to a severely self-limiting concept.

For many people, the first step to knowing who you are is to know who you are not. Almost all of the other answers to the question "Who are you?" are attempts to describe some aspect of what we do, the roles we play or how we appear. "I am this" or "I am that" are inherently dubious answers that may or may not be true. "*I am*" is truth.

Why is this discussion so important? What could we gain from asking ourselves who we are when we have so many pressing things in life to attend to? The answer is complex, but not hard to understand. Every decision you make in life is based on one of more assumptions that you have either made or, more likely, adopted from others and safely embedded in your subconscious as your map of the world. Bringing these questions to a conscious level for discussion allows us to reassess and reevaluate what serves us and what does not. So, here is a key: **when we choose to govern ourselves from a place of Consciousness, we reduce the likelihood that others will govern us from our subconscious.** If we are going to take back our power, understanding how and to whom we gave away that power is imperative. We have vested our power in others, including professionals, so-called experts and authorities, institutions and symbols, believing that these outside figures would serve us. As we begin to reclaim that power, we begin to change how we relate to our world. Gradually, we move from reacting to the events of our lives to responding and relating to these events. We stop being a consumer and start becoming what we came into this life to be: a creator! We move from the position of victim in life to master of our experiences. But note that being a master of our experiences is not the same concept as being able to control the events of life. There is a vast difference between the two. How we experience events and people depends greatly on our internal programming and perspective.

As you ponder these issues, you will realize that knowing who you are is fundamentally important to making sound decisions in life, especially in matters that pertain to your health.

Consider the questions below as you begin to get to know the real you.

1. Do you consider yourself to be a biological life form that came into being at birth and will cease to exist at the point of death?

2. Do you consider yourself to be a spirit or soul that lives in a physical, living body?

3. Do you consider yourself to be a spirit or soul that is having a physical experience in a temporal, 3-D world?

4. Do you believe that your spirit is temporal or that it exists beyond the confines of this physical life span?

5. Where were you before you came into this physical life?

6. Where will you go after this physical life?

7. Did you come into this life with a purpose?

8. Do you possess unique gifts, talents, aptitudes and abilities?

9. Have you identified those gifts, talents and abilities so that you can develop and share them in your life?

10. Do you know other people that appear to have unique gifts, talents, aptitudes and abilities?

11. Do you believe there is more to life than being forced to work in commerce most of your waking days in order to acquire a lot of stuff?

12. Is acquiring a lot of stuff an important goal in your life?

13. What things could you be without and still be you?

14. How many things could you be without and still be you?

15. Do you believe that acquiring a lot of stuff will provide happiness and contentment?

16. Do you feel a strong need to fit in with the ideas and opinions of others?

17. Are you here in this physical world to work and live subordinated to the directions and guidance of other people?

18. Are you capable of exercising sound and responsible judgment to direct your own life?

19. Do you feel you need the government or other authority to act as your parent and protector?

20. Do you believe you have the right to make mistakes?

21. Do you feel that you need to be protected from all the unpleasant possibilities in life?

22. Do you believe you need to be told by others what foods you can and cannot eat?

23. Do you believe that your judgment about which types of health or medical treatments you may choose for yourself or your family is inferior to the judgment of others?

24. Do you believe that other people should have the right to prohibit you from pursuing the healthcare choices that you deem best for you?

25. Do you believe that you should have the power and autonomy to make your own decisions about what to eat and how you treat your body, even if they are not always the best ones?

26. Do you believe that you should be able to search out and consult any form of medical or health treatment modality, even if it is not approved by the discipline currently in power?

At this moment, you may not be able to supply answers to many or even any of these questions. If so, that is perfectly okay. The fact that you have placed them into conscious thought is what matters. A big part of breaking through our old limitations in thought and perception is frequently *unlearning* what we have already been taught. Albert Einstein summed it up succinctly in saying: "The only thing that interferes with my learning is my education."

Chapter 4

Escaping from the Three M's

One might ask what this exercise in self-examination can be expected to achieve. After all, does it really matter whether we, as individual men and women, have any realistic handle on these seemingly esoteric questions? Does it make any difference in your health or the quality of your life? I would suggest that it can make all the difference not only in how you view the life experience, but also in how you approach the many decisions you are called upon to make each day, including those decisions that pertain to your health.

It has been said that if you don't believe in something, you will fall for anything. Having an understanding of who you are will act as an anchor for your passage through the turbulent seas of life. How?

Today's sophisticated technology allows us to easily track where people go, what they say and what they do. If that weren't enough, some people have developed a strange, insatiable desire to tell complete strangers the most intimate details of their lives and relationships through the advent of social media, such as Twitter, Facebook and the like. While the mere collection of information may or may not be viewed as an immediate problem, the reality is that information is power, the power to **Mold**, **Manipulate**, and **Manage** your life.

When skillfully done, most people will never know they have been manipulated. Most people are unaware of how their brain works, how their own perceptions are shaped, where their emotions come from and why they think or react the way they do toward certain events. But there are those who *do* understand how the mind works and how emotions and feelings are generated. Albert Einstein acknowledged the issue when he stated: "Few are those who see with their own eyes and feel with their own hearts."

Without the process of awakening, most people are no match for the super-sophisticated marketing and propaganda techniques used today. Yes, it's easy to spot the paid advertisement for what it is, but can you see the marketing and manipulation in the nightly news, government announcements, movies, classrooms and textbooks?

When you are manipulated sufficiently, your life and your expectations end up being managed. In order for you to make decisions in a manner consistent with the powers that be, your opinions need to be molded. This process has been going on for decades, and many of the things you currently believe are not beliefs that you fashioned yourself from your own information or experiences. If your information is limited (such as by careful editing and controlled access) or filtered (as in overt or covert censorship), you will not be privy to the spectrum of facts, data, opinions, research or experiences that could impact or change your resulting belief.

One of the greatest casualties resulting from the manipulation of information and your thinking is the suppression and diminishment of *your sense of the possible*! If you have no other sense of what is possible as an *alternative* to what you have been told, then you will likely believe what you were told. You adopt a severely limited view, giving you a frame of reference that causes you to immediately dismiss any new information that comes along as impossible or not credible. In effect, you have been conditioned to censor yourself, keeping your viewpoint diminished and your options severely limited. For example, what if I told you that there is an herbal cure for cancer? You would likely respond, "I don't believe it! If that were true, I would have heard about it!" Or, what if I said that certain energy therapies, such as EFT, have shown themselves to be highly successful in alleviating Post-Traumatic Stress Disorder. Most people would reply, "Energy therapy? That sounds too 'out there' for me. My doctor says an SSRI is the way to go." This form of control is much more elegant and efficient than chains and shackles. Control is the forerunner of dependence, and dependence is antithetical to strength, autonomy, freedom, health, wealth and especially critical thinking.

The media is quite adept at creating and molding public opinion. Some would argue that the creation of public opinion and your opinion is the primary goal of modern media, which has abandoned true, objective journalistic reporting for goal-directed content. "All the news that's fit to print," the motto of the *New York Times*, speaks boldly to their claim of authority to censure the news they deem "not fit" to print. Abraham Lincoln described the depth of the media's power well when he said, "In this and like communities, public sentiment is everything. With public sentiment, nothing can fail; without it, nothing can succeed. Consequently he who molds public sentiment goes deeper than he who enacts statutes or pronounces decisions."

For those who still vest any credibility in conventional media sources (what has been commonly called "main-stream" television, print media and radio), you are gently and relentlessly educated and influenced as to how you should view your world. Directly or indirectly, you are told:

- which news sources are trustworthy and which are not;
- what so-called public opinion currently is and what it is not;
- which political candidates are legitimate and electable and which are not;
- which points of view are reasonable and which are crazy;

- who the enemy is;
- which group of people you should fear;
- who you should hate;
- who is protecting you;
- who to admire and who to ignore;
- to talk about the virtues of so-called democracy rather than freedom;
- which medical treatments are valid and which are supposedly unproven;
- what is supposedly scientific and what is not;
- that Big Pharma medicine is based on science and natural therapies are not;
- that your genes control your health;
- that being on medication for life is normal;
- that eggs are good; no, wait a minute… eggs are bad;
- that access to medical services is a right;
- that government costs are not expenses; they are investments;
- that there are two sides to every issue, when in fact there may be multiple sides you will never hear about;
- that when there are two divergent points of view, the so-called truth is somewhere in between;
- whether the earth is warming or cooling;
- that men's ties should be wide or men's ties should be narrow;
- that button-down collars are "in" or button-down collars are "out";
- that women's hair should be short or women's hair should be long; and finally
- that if it was news, it would be reported.

This is how we are conditioned to think within the box, a box that was conceived, designed, defined, engineered and maintained by those who exert great influence within a society. The power and importance of manipulating the thoughts and beliefs of a people has long been recognized and is actively used today.

Let's look for a moment at the media in the United States. In 1983, 50 companies owned 90% of all media. In 2011–2012, that same 90% was owned by six corporations: Comcast, News-Corp, Disney, Viacom, CBS and Time Warner. According to some media analysts, this distribution of power means that approximately 235 media executives control what 275 million Americans see, read, hear and consider important. Perhaps we know why you can never find much to watch on television, even if you click through a couple hundred channels.

Chapter 5

The Power of Symbols

"Words are but symbols for the relations of things to one another and to us; nowhere do they touch upon absolute truth." – Friedrich Nietzsche

Our thinking, feelings and decisions are most easily manipulated through the careful use of symbols. Without a doubt, words are symbols, but so are institutions, photographs, flags, money, your car and your home, along with concepts, such as wealth and power. The names of diseases are symbols, too. Certainly, words have a shared dictionary definition that provides a basis for communication. Some words may have multiple dictionary meanings, and people may misunderstand or disagree based on which meaning they are using. But the real power of symbols is experienced at the subconscious level, where an emotional meaning, feeling or association is attached to the word, image or idea. Thus, the power of the symbol is often *felt* more than *thought*. So, ask yourself the following:

>What do you *feel* when you think of the word "wealthy"?
>What do you *feel* when you see a Swastika?
>What do you *feel* when you see your country's flag?
>What do you *feel* when you see the US flag?
>What do you *feel* when you see a picture of the Eiffel Tower?
>What do you *feel* when you see a $100 dollar bill?

What do you *feel* when you see a Rolls Royce drive by?
What do you *feel* when you hear the phrase "You have cancer"?
What do you *feel* when someone calls you a "dog"?

All of these items are simply words, and although the words may have multiple meanings, they are merely symbols of those meanings. Through the use of symbols, your feelings and, by extension, your thinking and decisions can be (and are) manipulated.

In its most innocent form, the effort put forth to convince you to purchase a product or service is called advertising. Generally, advertising is designed to create a sense of need where none previously existed. If the form of conditioning that we call advertising did not work, then small businesses, major corporations and governments would not spend billions of dollars trying to convince you of something. Advertising *does* work, and people can be motivated to purchase things they never knew existed and do not even need. Advertising can be subtle, obvious, obnoxious, soft sell, hard sell and subliminal.

When an *idea* is being sold rather than a product, and the origin of the effort is a government, that form of manipulation is referred to as propaganda. Propaganda is simply political advertising designed to sell you an idea. The Wikipedia definition is:

> **Propaganda** is a form of communication that is aimed at influencing the attitude of a community toward some cause or position. Propaganda is usually repeated and dispersed over a wide variety of media in order to create the desired result in audience attitudes.

The promoted idea could be to support a war, a bailout program, a political candidate, a political cause or any of a number of other ideas, projects or causes. The movie *Wag the Dog* is a contemporary movie that illustrates the art of propaganda as utilized by governments today.

The father of modern advertising and propaganda was undoubtedly Edward Bernays. Bernays was a nephew of Sigmund Freud and may have been the first modern figure to synthesize advertising with psychology. He is also noted for his practice of using the supposedly unbiased authority of third parties to convince others of the credibility of the advertised message. These techniques were immensely successful.

When the tobacco industry wanted to expand cigarette sales by getting more women to smoke, they hired Edward Bernays. At that time, the 1930s, it was pretty much taboo (either legally or socially) for women to smoke cigarettes openly in public. Women who did smoke were only allowed to do so in private or in designated smoking places for women, and those caught smoking in public could be arrested. Bernays cleverly staged events in which women defiantly smoked in public and redefined the cigarettes they smoked as "Torches of Freedom." These staged events were picked up by the news media, which provided free publicity. The campaign was wildly successful. Ultimately, the taboo was broken and women were now socially permitted to get lung cancer in equal opportunity to men.

Another important campaign involved The Aluminum Company of America (ALCOA) and their desire to find a way sell off their fluoride as a beneficial substance. Fluoride was an abundant, toxic by-product of aluminum processing that was difficult to dispose of. Bernays was hired to help convince people and the state that fluoride would help prevent tooth decay. To do so, he brought the in American Dental Association as a so-called third-party expert to validate the promotion. The campaign worked, and Alcoa could gradually sell off its fluoride to water treatment facilities all around the United States and make a profit. Although not everyone was convinced of the safety or efficacy of total body fluoridation, enough people in positions of power made it appear as fact. It was only in the last decade that the real story of fluoride has emerged with sufficient new evidence to rebuke the original fluoride story.

Bernays was a genius, and it did not take long for the US government to take note of his ability to convince people to accept ideas they had formerly rejected. Bernays eventually helped the US government promote various wars and government campaigns to the American people. He also was behind the recommendation to change the name of the War Department to the Department of Defense.

Bernays believed that his method of public manipulation was justified. In his 1928 book, *Propaganda*, Bernays argued for the scientific manufacture of public opinion, saying:

> The conscious and intelligent manipulation of the organized habits and opinions of the masses is an important element in democratic society. Those who manipulate this unseen mechanism of society constitute an invisible government which is the true ruling power of our country... We are governed, our minds are molded, our tastes formed, our ideas suggested, largely by men we have never heard of. ...

Bernays goes on to say that in almost every aspect of our daily lives, "whether in the sphere of politics or business, in our social conduct or our ethical thinking, we are dominated by the relatively small number of persons... It is they who pull the wires which control the public mind".

In most Western societies, opinion molding is accomplished through elegant and sophisticated measures while maintaining the appearance of a free press. Typically, the press serves large corporate and government interests in exchange for favor and privilege.

But while making such a statement is rather easy, it denies you a feeling for the depth and breadth of the evidence upon which such a conclusion has been made. Since a key concept in Mind Myths is that personal liberation comes from making our own decisions rather than merely accepting those offered by others, I will present a number of important quotations here and in upcoming sections for your thoughtful consideration rather then ask you to simply accept my conclusions. The figure below illustrates how little separation there is between those who control media and those who control government.

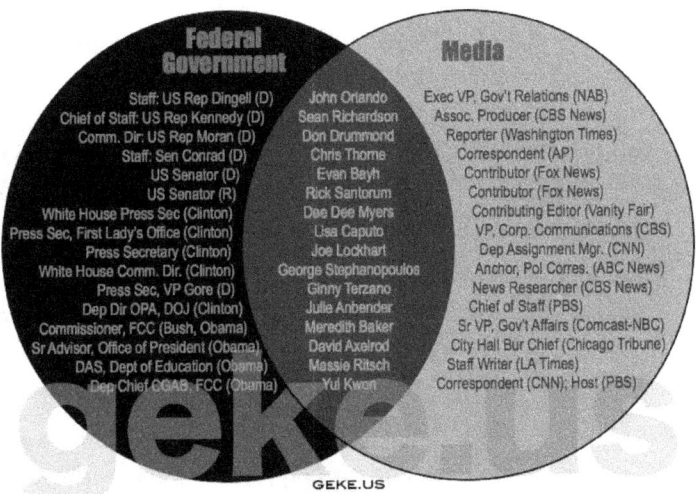

Figure 1: Overlap Between Media and US Federal Government (used with permission, http://geke.us)

Noam Chomsky, an American linguist, philosopher and professor emeritus in the Department of Linguistics & Philosophy at MIT, shared this insight:

> The smart way to keep people passive and obedient is to strictly limit the spectrum of acceptable opinion, but allow very lively debate within that spectrum - even encourage the more critical and dissident views. That gives people the sense that there's free thinking going on, while all the time the

presuppositions of the system are being reinforced by the limits put on the range of the debate.

Professor Carroll Quigley of Georgetown University had this to say in his book, *Tragedy and Hope: A History of The World in Our Time*;

> "...the elements of choice and freedom may survive for the ordinary individual in that he may be free to make a choice between two opposing political groups (even if these groups have little policy choice within the parameters of policy established by the experts)..... But, in general, his freedom and choice will be controlled within very narrow alternatives by the fact that he will be numbered from birth and followed, as a number, through his educational training, his required military or other public service, his tax contributions, his health and medical requirements, and his final retirement and death benefits.

Professor Quigley continues by saying that the two parties should represent opposing policies and principles from the Right and the Left, "...is a foolish idea acceptable only to the doctrinaire and academic thinkers. Instead, the two parties should be almost identical, so that the American people can 'throw the rascals out' at any election without leading to any profound or extreme shifts in policy".

Aldous Huxley made this comment in the preface to his book *Brave New World*:

> The greatest triumphs of propaganda have been accomplished, not by doing something, but by refraining from doing. Great is truth, but still greater, from a practical point of view, is silence about truth. By simply not mentioning certain subjects, by lowering what Mr. Churchill calls an 'iron curtain' between the masses and such facts or arguments as the local political

> bosses regard as undesirable, totalitarian propagandists have influenced opinion much more effectively than they could have done by the most eloquent denunciations, the most compelling of logical rebuttals.

All governments, from democracies to dictatorships employ propaganda to achieve their goals. Hitler's Minster of Propaganda, Herman Goering, had this to say:

> Why of course the people don't want war. Why should some poor slob on a farm want to risk his life in a war when the best he can get out of it is to come back to his farm in one piece? Naturally the common people don't want war: neither in Russia, nor in England, nor for that matter in Germany. That is understood. But after all it is the leaders of a country who determine the policy and it is always a simple matter to drag the people along, whether it is a democracy or fascist dictatorship, or a parliament or a communist dictatorship. Voice or no voice, the people can always be brought to the bidding of the leaders. That is easy. All you have to do is tell them they are being attacked, and denounce the peace makers for lack of patriotism and exposing the country to danger. It works the same in any country.

In the more sophisticated forms of opinion management, events, circumstances, discussions and facts can be created, edited and orchestrated so that the reaction that arises from the target audience was not only predictable, but also desirable to the manipulator. Thus, the opinions, conclusions and beliefs that you create about such events or issues genuinely feel as if they were the product of your own thoughtful analysis. But in reality, since most of the information you received was controlled and presented in such a specific and coordinated manner, there were few other conclusions you could have reached. That may sound incredible, but people's reactions are somewhat predictable when events and information are properly staged. Create a banking crisis. Create crime on the streets. Create an oil crisis. Create a war. As people experience pain, frustration and fear, they cry out for someone to fix the problem, and those who orchestrated the crisis just happen to have the solution prepared and ready!

Chapter 6

Creating Opinion By Creating Crises

The method most commonly used for the creation of opinion or political force is called Hegelian dialectics, named after 19th-Century German philosopher and theologian Georg Wilhelm Friedrich Hegel (1770–1831), who wrote *The Science of Logic* in 1812. Although the technique has been used for thousands of years, the Hegelian dialectic is a framework for guiding people's thoughts and actions into a conflict that ultimately leads to a predetermined solution. It is manipulation on a grand scale. It consists of three parts or steps: thesis, antithesis and synthesis, which are more popularly referred to as problem, reaction and solution. First, someone or some group creates the problem. Once established, opposition (or the appearance of opposition) to the problem must be generated. Lastly, a so-called solution is offered to resolve the original problem. Typically, in this process, the same people who created the problem in the first place offer up and vigorously support a solution, either directly or through associates. Political groups and governments have used this framework for decades, but it is only effective when people are *unaware* of its use. Only certain solutions are ever discussed to resolve social, financial, political or governmental crises, because those crises serve to move public sentiment to where it was intended to go. Need support for a massively expensive and unpopular program? Need to restrict personal liberties? Easy. Just create a new enemy or launch a new war. Need to sell a new vaccine that is profitable but potentially risky? Just create a scare about a possible global pandemic and people will clamor for your solution. Using the principles of Hegel, people will ask for the very solutions they would have opposed under different circumstances. Once you understand how this system works, you will notice it being used almost constantly by the media, social engineers and government policymakers.

How is this possible? Well, developmental biologists and neuroscientists recognize that certain portions of the brain are responsible for very basic responses, such as fear. In what used to be referred to as the reptilian brain, our limbic system is where we perceive and react to potential threats to our safety. This part of the brain can also be conditioned with certain responses or become hypersensitive to certain situations or conditions, as in Post-Traumatic Stress Disorder.

When we become fearful, our higher cortical thinking functions become impaired and our ability to make sound, rational decisions is also impaired. We *react* to things out of fear, rather than *respond* from a position of careful thought. You can witness this kind of shock and fear on the face of a newly diagnosed cancer patient as they learn the news of their condition. While experiencing such a state of shock is hardly the time to make good, clear decisions that serve your best interests.

All governments and political powers have used war, the specter of terrorism or some other threat from bad guys to create fear in their population. The medical system also employs fear when you talk with your physician about the possibility of not following their recommendations and going the so-called alternative route. At this point, you will likely hear a litany of awful consequences that could befall you or your child if you do not follow their recommendations. Fear opens the door for compliance and control. Our reaction, generated through our experience of fear, justified or not, impairs our rational thinking abilities as well as access to our higher intuitive abilities. We become ensnared in fight-or-flight survival mode of and there is little room for more.

But due to this global awakening, people are increasingly motivated to ask questions, do their own research and put less trust in so-called experts. Evidence of this trend is poking through here and there, such as the poll conducted on the Oswald/Kennedy murders in the US in 1962. In a 2009 CBS Poll, by a 74 percent to 13 percent margin, the American public said that they believe there was an official cover-up in the investigation to prevent the truth from being disclosed. Why did people not just accept the conclusions from the government-sponsored experts? When you ask those non-believers, you will likely find that each of them made some effort to investigate the facts behind the headlines and what they read did not make sense.

Our ancestral distrust of other tribes can also be exploited by the creation of a threat and giving it a face. Hitler did this effectively in Germany, and millions of people suffered and died as a result. The creation of a boogeyman, whether domestic or foreign, is a time-proven and effective strategy.

Tribal conflicts and the us-versus-them emotional pattern are further exploited and strengthened through the promotion of innocent events, such as regional sports, which provide an amplified outlet for ancient tribal rivalry and competition. While many people enjoy sports for entertainment, being a fan has morphed into an identity and obsession for millions. It has always bewildered me why privately owned, for-profit businesses, such as a regional baseball team or football team in the US, are the recipients of free television advertising that all other privately owned businesses have to pay for! Employees in banks can wear the jersey of their favorite team when the play-offs approach, but I dare say they would not be allowed to wear a jersey promoting their brother-in-law's electrical contracting business. Why the double standard? This custom may depend a lot more on which ideas and values are being fostered than on money and profits.

Part III

The Power of Perspective

Chapter 7

Creating Our Perspective

> "All our knowledge has its origins in our perceptions." - Leonardo da Vinci

Beginning with the earliest years of our lives, we learn from those around us and start to form our mental map of our world, our perception of what we call reality. This map is our internal, personal ideal of how life is, how the world works and how we interact with it in order to get our needs met. We all have such a map, and it can both help and hinder us depending on whether we are willing to update it periodically.

Developmental biologists tell us that, until the age of six or seven, we accept everything we see, hear and experience as literally true. Ideas do not go through any sort of conscious intellectual filter that permits us to accept or reject them. This includes, of course, both verbal and nonverbal experiences. Any parent will tell you that kids are very perceptive and tuned in to their parents and what is going on around them, even if parents sometimes think (or hope) they are not. Thus, the actions and attitudes of parents toward matters involving food, mealtime, illness, pain and crises serve as the model blueprint for the child's personal map of their world. For example, the use of sweet foods as a reward for good behavior, good grades or other apparently positive events may seem both harmless and productive. However, it teaches children that a link exists between certain behaviors and receiving a reward. Could this be the reason why so many Americans use food or drink for reward and for escape? Do young minds interpret their loving grandmother bringing cakes or pies when she visited as a message that love and acceptance is intimately tied to sweets? If the grandmother had brought carrot sticks upon visiting, would the same emotional link have been created? Behaviors that appear beneficial in early life are not always so later in life. Renowned Swiss psychologist and psychiatrist Carl Jung illustrated this point when he said: "....we cannot live the afternoon of life according to the program of life's morning; for what was great in the morning will be little at evening, and what in the morning was true will at evening have become a lie."

As humans, we appear to be hardwired with a need to know. Our mind is filled with questions that inspire our search for answers. Why did that happen? What did I do to deserve that? Why did I develop fibromyalgia? Our need to explain and understand the events and happenings in our personal world, and our larger world, compels us to seek answers. Not knowing creates anxiety and uneasiness, as if we expect our world to always follow a logical and orderly process. To satisfy this hunger, our mind can do one of three things:

1) we can ask questions directed toward discovering the truth;
2) we can accept the assumptions and conclusions offered by various external sources, such as the media, experts, physicians, etc.; or
3) we can create assumptions in our mind that will just as easily satisfy our need to know, even if they are totally untrue.

Ironically, whether the answers to our questions are true or not appears to be less important to the mind than having an answer at all. This is why most people prefer to see what they wish to see and hear what they want to hear. They have already accepted or created an answer, and they believe 100% in what they believe. To one degree or another, we have all done this. These assumptions become the threads that weave the fabric of our map of reality, our own personal book of rules and explanations that we consult thousands of times each day. When new information or questions arise, we consult our rulebook and judge the new fact or information accordingly.

In fact, you need only look at most high school history books to realize the scope of the conditioning. Mainstream history books tend to present history as a nice, neat package of mostly linear progress and achievement from roughly 3100 BC to the present. The present, of course, is presented as the absolute pinnacle of human progress and the flower of achievement. After all, just look at all the neat gadgets and technology that we have. If you visit Stonehenge in the south of England, you will see a depiction of the creators of this incredible megalithic site as a band of primitive knuckle-draggers. But no one wants to explain how these supposed primitives quarried and moved the huge inner bluestones from the Preseli Mountains in southwest Wales (some 168 miles away) to the Stonehenge site. Nor does anyone explain how they raised the nine-ton lintel pieces atop the Sarsen stones without the benefit of modern cranes used today. You only have to do an Internet search on Gobekli Tepi in Turkey (now dated to be 12,000 years old), research the vast sunken cities off the coast of India and Japan (dated 9,500 years old) or visit the ruins at Machu Picchu, the lost city of the Inca in Peru (of unknown age) to realize that ours is not the first civilization to be here, nor the most accomplished. Yet for all of the incredible *tangible* history represented by this forbidden archaeology, these marvels are simply omitted from conventional history books. (An excellent review of this archaeology and history is *Commonwealth* by Freddy Silva.)

What we fail to realize and what we do not wish to examine is that most of the so-called facts or truths in our book of reality are actually illusions, myths and lies. But because having knowledge helps to make us feel safer in an uncertain and bewildering world, we defend our knowledge even when it is wrong. This tendency, of course, quickly becomes a trap. As humans, we create our assumptions to explain what we do not understand and then let the assumptions control our decisions and our lives. In matters of health and disease, doing so can be deadly. This tendency is well illustrated by Leo Tolstoy's observation that even for those people who are adept at handling problems of the "greatest complexity", they "can seldom accept even the simplest and most obvious truth if it be such as would oblige them to admit the falsity of conclusions which they have delighted in explaining to colleagues, which they have proudly taught to others, and which they have woven, thread by thread, into the fabric of their lives.

Over the years, I have read countless self-help books about "taking your power back". This idea is emotionally attractive, since it speaks to a sense shared by many people that they live a life without much control. Having more personal power would imply that you would have more control, right? But in so many of those books, just how one went about accomplishing that was never clearly articulated. Take my power back? What does that mean? Just how do I do that? Where did I put my power in the first place? Did I lose it? Did I give it away? How much power do I really have anyway?

It has become abundantly clear over the years that reclaiming one's power is, in fact, possible, but not necessarily in the way that I first believed. And we do not necessarily gain more control over our lives by doing so. Control in life is, I believe, an illusion. At best, we can steer our lives by the choices we make, but we cannot really get control. I gained insight into this question through the course of thousands of one-on-one consultations with clients who were seeking answers to their own health-related questions. Whether their issue was migraines, ulcerative colitis, fibromyalgia, asthma or any of a dozen other chronic conditions, the underlying generic issues relating to becoming well all appeared to be surprisingly similar. The more patients attempted to exert control over their lives, the more stressed and frustrated they became. They held a strong idea of how life should be. Years ago, I heard a definition of stress that I think is extremely useful. Stress can be defined as "the distance between where you are in life and where you think you should be."

Stress, then, arises from a *perception* and a *judgment*.

Chapter 8

An Act of Surrender

It is axiomatic in clinical nutrition that before you will change what you eat, you will need to change how you think. When you change how you think about food, life, nourishment, short-term vs. long-term consequences and sensory gratification, you will easily and willingly change how you eat. This change usually begins when a client translates a recommended dietary change into a question such as, "So, I have to give up grains and gluten?" Lurking just below the surface of this question is the conscious or subconscious fear of being deprived. After all, having to give up something that you have enjoyed for many years certainly sounds like a sacrifice. In Western society, we do not do "giving up" very well. Inevitably, this sense of making a sacrifice stems from how we relate to food and perhaps even a belief that we should be able to eat whatever we want and still enjoy perfect health. Is that true? Where did that assumption come from? Who created it? What was the question that this assumption was created to satisfy?

In these discussions, it is important to recognize the real issue and examine what we hold to be true. In the foregoing example, the gluten-sensitive person who is now *aware* that avoiding gluten is a necessary step in their journey back to good health has a choice in how they view their situation. They may choose to view the elimination of gluten as a sacrifice and deprivation. Or, they may choose to view the elimination of gluten as an *exchange*: a surrender of one thing (in this case, eating gluten-containing foods) in exchange for receiving something of equal or greater value (better health, reduced symptoms, etc.). Either way, the act of avoiding all gluten-containing foods and the resulting relief from the symptoms provoked by ingesting gluten is a matter of cause and effect. But which attitude will better serve the patient over the long term? How long do you think the patient who feels deprived and resents their elimination of gluten will stay with the healthier choice? By consciously reframing this experience as an act of deliberate choice that provides benefits and rewards greater than the act of surrendering that food, we can effectively neutralize the frustration and resentment we might feel toward making the healthier choice.

The collaboration described above is in stark contrast to the old medical model in which physician and patient often acted out the roles of parent and child. In the past, a patient might have said, "The doctor told me I can't eat wheat" or "I hope you are not angry with me Doctor Jones; I was bad, and I cheated on my diet." When we think in these terms, we have given away our power to another person (the physician), a belief system (the allopathic medical model) and a dynamic based on reward and punishment. Whether you "cheat" on your diet or not, the only person who will suffer or gain is *you*. Who did you cheat? Who suffered as a result?

There are a number of phrases I have heard from clients that signify a surrender of their personal power:

- My doctor put me on an acid-blocker drug;
- My doctor told me I can't eat wheat;
- I don't know what this medication is for, but the doctor told me to take it;
- My doctor said I am depressed and need medication;
- My doctor said there are no side effects from this medication;
- My doctor said there is no cure for this condition. I just have to live with it;
- If it weren't safe, it wouldn't be on the market;

- The package said there were "zero" trans fats, so I guess it means there are no trans fats in the product;
- We are all overweight in my family. It's genetic and I can't do much about it;
- What can you expect for being 50 years old? and
- It's natural and normal to get arthritis when you are older.

There are hundreds of assumptions and beliefs that we have either created ourselves or accepted from others that define how we think about our bodies and our health. Some are extremely subtle and lurk more secretively in the subconscious mind, while others are profound and known to our conscious mind. Many are illusions, if innocuous, and lies when deadly. The courage to ask the critical questions and reexamine what we think is true is frequently the deciding issue for whether a person recovers from a serious or chronic disabling illness or condition. Continuing to live in the prison of ideas and beliefs that lead to the creation of the condition is unlikely to provide an answer.

When you examine the sometimes miraculous stories of people who overcame serious, life-threatening cancers or burns, the central element in their recovery was a realignment of their thinking processes and beliefs. Many recovered after jettisoning their old lifestyles and accumulated anger and resentment. Others decided to "follow their bliss" and made drastic life changes in the expectation of only having a few months to live; yet, ten years later, are still living and enjoying life, much to the amazement of the medical community. Healing is healing, and it is always a mind-body experience. For many, the road to healing may hold profound spiritual elements as well. We must learn to distinguish between the process of healing and treating a condition. Treating a specific, medically named collection of symptoms with the intention of controlling or reducing symptoms is another matter entirely.

Chapter 9

Recalibrating Our Perceptions

"The trouble with the world is not that people know too little, but that they know so many things that just aren't so."
– Mark Twain

Changing our perspective on an issue can frequently make all the difference in the world in how we see it. Although we do not usually take the time to do so, we have the ability whenever we choose. For example, it might be easy to judge the poor and inattentive service of the early morning breakfast waitress until we learn that she has been awake all night with a sick child and works two jobs as a single mom. Suddenly, no tip as punishment for the poor service is transformed into an extra tip due to her personal circumstances. Unfortunately, we do not always get the other side of the story in life, so we draw our conclusions and make our judgments based on incomplete information, which we filter through our perceptions.

Fortunately, there are other ways we can challenge the truthfulness of our perceptions. One way is to turn to examples in science, specifically physics, to help us view the world differently. We rely heavily on our physical senses of vision and hearing to process our experiences in the world. Based on the information we gather from our very limited five senses, we conclude that we live in a three-dimensional world where people and things appear to be separate, where things appear to be solid and where time moves in only one direction. In fact, we are quite literally prisoners of our limited sensory capacities.

The human bias is to exclusively believe our five senses. If we cannot sense something (by hearing, seeing, tasting, feeling or smelling), then we act as if it does not exist. So, look around you now. Squint and look very carefully. Can you see the radio and television signals that are all around you right now? They are passing right through you, see? Can you hear the waves of ultraviolet light streaming down from the sun and that cause your skin to tan or burn? Can you feel gravity keeping your feet securely planted on the earth? Could you see, taste, touch or feel the x-rays emitted from the CT scanner when you had your sinus CT scan?

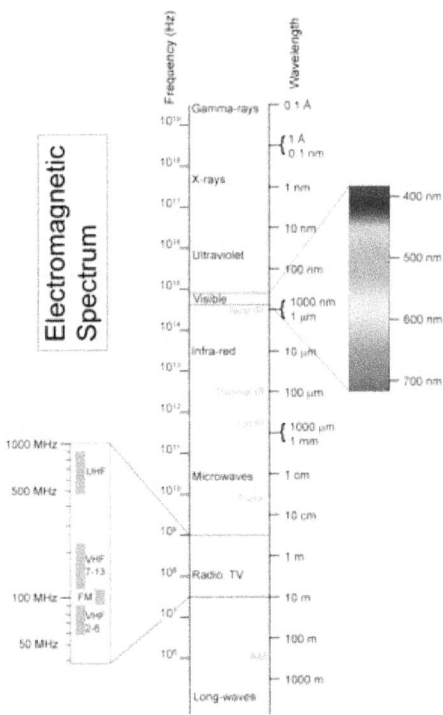

Figure 2: The Electromagnetic Spectrum: The Visible and Invisible (from Creative Commons/Wikipedia/Wikimedia Commons)

45

Our hearing is limited to a range of frequencies that we refer to as the audible frequency range. It is typically defined as those frequencies between 20 and 20,000 cycles per second (called Hertz), although considerable variation exists from one human to another. Considering the vast world of frequencies, this range is very narrow. As a result, man has designed and built equipment that can pick up the many other frequencies not detectable to our ears or senses. The typical frequency range dogs can detect is roughly 40 to 60,000 Hertz, with variation based on the breed and age of the dog. Thus your dog can hear many sounds that are real but beyond your hearing range, such as a dog whistle. Bats can hear frequencies between 20 and 120,000 Hertz. Bottlenose dolphins, meanwhile, can detect a range typically between 0.25 and 150,000 Hertz. They use the higher frequencies for echolocation purposes. The point is that our sense of hearing is limited even compared to other living species on earth. In terms of the cosmos, humans are nearly deaf.

As humans, we say we "hear" when vibrational waves that are carried through the air are funneled into our ear canals and hit a thin membrane we call the eardrum. As the eardrum moves in response to these vibrational waves, it in turn causes the three middle ear bones (the malleus, incus and stapes) to move and displace fluid in the cochlea or inner ear. The moving fluid causes small hairs to also move, thus creating the electrical signals that our brain picks up and decodes as sounds. Complicated, isn't it? With all of the steps involved, it is a wonder that we can hear at all!

But here is the point of this brief biology discussion. Our ears are simply transducers of vibrational information. Said differently, you have never heard a single word spoken in your entire life! No, not one word! What you have "heard" are specific vibrational patterns that were collected and transmitted by a complex group of biological structures and eventually interpreted by your brain as a pattern. We have all agreed that certain patterns constitute a particular word. The vibrational pattern of the word "apple" is a different vibrational pattern than that created by the song of a chickadee or that created by a bell. With learning and training, our brains can distinguish one pattern from the other. The difficulties we experience in vibrational pattern recognition can be demonstrated quite nicely when you are trying to learn a foreign language. I know and understand only a handful of words in Spanish, and when I visit a Spanish-speaking country and listen to native Spanish-speaking people, my brain cannot identify or distinguish the vibrational patterns that we refer to as "Spanish words". With effort, I can learn to do so. But I am never hearing a "word".

Let's look at vision (pardon the pun). The human eye can detect vibrational frequencies within a very narrow frequency range: between 390 nm and 750 nm or so, depending on the age and health of the eye. Defined in terms of frequency, this corresponds to a band in the vicinity of 400–790 THz (which is called Terahertz and is equal to 10^{12} Hertz or 1,000,000,000,000 Hz.) We call this the visible spectrum because these are the wavelengths we can see, of course. But it is a tiny slice of a vastly larger spectrum of frequencies that we cannot detect. When the rods and cones in the retina of the human eye are stimulated by vibrational frequencies within the visible light spectrum, electrical signals are created and channeled to the brain via the optic nerve. (By the way, we do not see with our eyes. We "see" by using a complex decoding system in our brain. We *sense* with our eyes. The visual cortex at the back of the brain is where our brain decodes the nerve impulse information received via the optic nerve and creates the images that we "see".) So, when the retina is exposed to vibrational frequencies between 526 and 606 THz (or as defined by wavelength, 495–570 nm), we "see" the color we have all agreed to call "green". When the rods and cones of the retina are stimulated by those vibrational frequencies between 631 and 668 THz (or 450–475 nm), we "see" the color we agree to call "blue". It is the same with other frequencies within the visible spectrum. When the rods and cones of the retina are stimulated by frequencies outside of this narrow band of frequencies, we do not see anything. What are we not seeing?

This discussion raises the question of what is real and how we define reality. This question was succinctly asked by the character Morpheus in the movie *The Matrix* when he asked Neo, "What is real? How do you define real? If you're talking about what you can feel, what you can smell, what you can taste and see, then real is simply electrical signals interpreted by your brain."

Our sensory decoding capabilities are also exquisitely vulnerable to distortion and even error. Sometimes, these experiences create innocent fun, as with various optical or visual illusions. Because of how our brains are designed to decode incoming signals, it is possible to "see" something that does not or cannot exist in the real world. The two examples below illustrate this point:

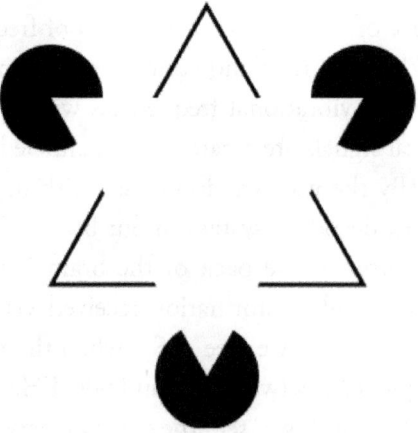

Figure 3: Kanizsa Triangle (from Wikimedia Commons, GNU Free Documentation, Creative Commons License)

When viewing the figure above, called the Kanizsa Triangle, the brain decodes the electrical signals received from the eyes and constructs a white triangle superimposed over the black triangle; however, no white triangle really exists. Most viewers also "see" the white triangle as being brighter than the adjacent white area of the paper, though such is not the case. The figure below is known as the Penrose Triangle. This optical illusion causes the brain to see an image of a three-dimensional object that *appears* to exist but is impossible to construct in our 3-D reality. There are thousands of additional examples of optical illusions that can trick our brain decoding system in one or more ways. But the point of all this fun is merely to illustrate how easy it is for us to misperceive and misinterpret the sensory information we gather.

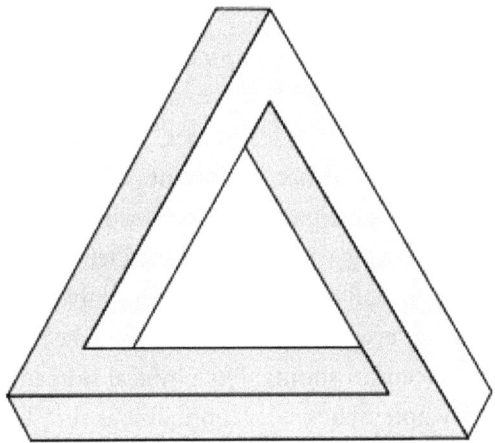

Figure 4: The Penrose Triangle, named after mathematician Roger Penrose. (Image adapted from Brandon Tran at 123opticalillusions.com)

Most of the objects that we see in our world do not create or emit light by themselves. Certainly the sun creates its own light as photons that stream to earth. The moon merely reflects the light from the sun. In the same way you see the moon, what you see when you look at a chair, car, tree or house is the light that is reflected by those objects according to its absorptive and reflective properties. You have never actually seen a chair, car, tree or house. Since the object did not create and emit its own light, you could only see that light which was reflected. Further, how do you know that your eyes and brain have decoded the vibrational frequencies reflected from those objects in exactly the same manner as your wife or brother or best friend? We all assume that we do, but can you ever know? Could someone see reds a little more intensely than you do? Or, perhaps you see blue as a slightly darker hue than your daughter does? And none of us see or process any of the other vibrational frequencies above or below the visible spectrum, even though we are literally bathed in these frequencies all the time: the AM and FM waves of radio, the higher frequency microwaves emitted by your cell phone and the x-rays and gamma rays emitted by stars, black holes and medical equipment. There is a whole world of energy and frequency patterns that we simply cannot detect with the limited sensitivity of our biological senses. Therefore, we live our lives as if they were not there or not important. Yet all of these different frequencies and vibrational patterns exist simultaneously in the same space without interfering with each other! Defined by our sense of sight, humans are virtually blind within this Universe and because of this limitation we see everything as distinctly separate. Albert Einstein illustrated this concept in stating: "As physical human beings, we are part of a greater whole that we conceptualize as the "Universe", but a part limited in time and space. We experience ourselves, our thoughts and feelings as something separate from the rest... This delusion is a kind of prison, restricting us to our personal desires and to affection for a few persons nearest to us. Our task must be to free ourselves from the prison by widening our circle of compassion to embrace all living creatures and the whole of nature in its beauty".

Chapter 10

Sound Creates Form

Experiments by Swiss scientist and medical doctor Dr. Hans Jenny (1904–1972) in the 1960s provided great insight into the relationship between sound (vibrational frequencies) and form. Dr. Jenny discovered that when he passed different frequencies through a metal plate upon which he had sprinkled an otherwise inert fine powder, such as fine sand, the particles would almost magically align into patterns unique to the frequency being used. The same frequency always produced the same pattern, so it was quite clear that the frequency conveyed specific information about structure to the particles and altered their relationship to each other. Some patterns were not only extremely complex, but also mimicked shapes found in nature and the universe. Even tones or words created by the human vocal cords were capable of generating a pattern.

This study is called cymatics, which is defined as the study of wave phenomena and vibration. Although the definition sounds dreadfully dull, it is anything but. You can easily search for "cymatics" on the web and locate a number of amazing videos that demonstrate this principle quite clearly. Two such web sites are www.cymaticsource.com and www.cymatics.org, where you can read more about cymatics and watch videos of this effect. Frequencies clearly impart information, and cymatics sheds light on the nature of the universe and how energy relates to form. Since everything is energy, the interconnectedness of all things begins to make sense.

As you can clearly see, cymatics demonstrates that sound (frequency) contains information and can create form. But we also know that the reverse is true: sound can destroy form. Some readers may be familiar with an older advertising campaign that utilized the voice of a famous female singer to shatter a glass in an effort to prove fidelity of reproduction using their recording tape. While a glass can be easily shattered with the right frequency, not everything around it also shattered. Therefore, the frequency is specific to the material selected. Another example of the effects of frequency and resonance at work is the collapse of the Tacoma Narrows Bridge in Washington State (USA), which collapsed on November 7, 1940 due to the resonant vibrations created by gale force winds.

When we begin to understand the magnitude of this phenomenon, we can begin to appreciate the impact that the frequencies represented by our words may have on our biology and that of others. Our thoughts are waveforms themselves, and so we begin to understand that a very real connection between the intangible energy of sound and the tangible response of matter exists. Of course, our perception that one form of energy is intangible while another is tangible is purely an artifact resulting from the severe limitations of our five sensory mechanisms.

Given the lack of information we collect through our biological five senses, the number of rigid and dogmatic judgments and conclusions we make about things, people and the world is astounding. There is so much that we cannot see and even more that we choose not to see. We then spend the rest of our time living as if what we do see is all that there is. However, as Albert Einstein pointed out, "Reality is merely an illusion, albeit a very persistent one."

Our limited 3-D perspective about reality is part of the reason why it is difficult to motivate people to address the inherent dangers of holding a cell phone up to their head. We simply cannot see, feel, hear, taste or otherwise sense the microwave radiation that is emitted from the antenna and how it affects our brain tissue. The fact that it may take years for the damage to appear makes the danger seem even more abstract given all the pressing issues we face each day. The limitation of our five senses is also one of the reasons why people often have difficulty accepting the concept of "energy healing". They cannot see it, measure it or understand how it works, so they prefer the "real" world of blood tests, x-rays, and drugs. Even though CT scanners utilize invisible energy as well, people will accept *that* energy because the medical system has endorsed it.

Speaking at a more eclectic level, what if there were whole populations of life forms whose frequencies were simply outside the range of our senses? Or, life forms that exist within one of the other dimensions that physicists know to exist, beyond our three dimensions plus time? What a rich universe it would be!

Chapter 11

A Rose by Any Other Name

Now that we have a willingness to temporarily alter our perceptions, let's turn our attention to food. As children, we were taught the names of various foods and could add new foods to our culinary experience as our language skills grew and we matured. For many people, the consumption of food is far removed from the raising, growing or preparing food for the market. Most of us do not grow our own crops, raise or "dress" our own chickens or milk cows and churn the cream into butter. Other people do that. If you are not a biologist, you may not have a good grasp of the taxonomy of foods, or how they are related botanically in families. For example, rice, wheat, oats, rye, corn and spelt are all "grasses" and thus are related to each other.

So what's in a name? To paraphrase Shakespeare, a rose by any other name is still a rose. But if we did change the name, would you feel differently about it?

Did you ever eat the moldy curds collected from a lactating bovid? Did you ever eat baked ovaries with cinnamon and walnuts? How about fungus? Do you like yours lightly sautéed in olive oil with onion?

You probably do, but not by those names.

The moldy curd collected from a lactating bovid is the milk collected from cows, to which bacteria or mold is added in order to produce cheese. Perhaps you are a connoisseur of a fine blue cheese, such as

Roquefort, gorgonzola or British stilton? Blue cheese is produced by adding the mold or the mold spores of *penicillium* to milk and then letting it ferment, usually in a temperature-controlled environment, such as a cave. The veins of blue, blue-gray or blue-green mold running through the cheese give it the unique and characteristic sharp taste. The unique smell of blue cheese is due to the bacteria *brevibacterium linens* which is the same bacteria that creates the smell we call "foot odor". Yummy. The terms "blue cheese" or "Roquefort" are, therefore, agreed upon name-symbols for this particular food; renaming the food conveniently allows us to side-step the less savory details.

Baked apples are a favorite dessert in colder, North American climates, and are often prepared with liberal amounts of cinnamon, walnuts, nutmeg or other spices and slowly baked until done. Delicious! Not an appetizing dish, though, if I change the word-symbol to the naked biology of an apple being an ovary. Baked ovaries, anyone? Thanks, I'll pass.

There are many edible mushrooms and some that are quite deadly. All mushrooms are, in fact, fungi. While some people enjoy the pastime of mushroom hunting, most people obtain this edible fungus by purchasing it at their grocery stores. However, few prefer to offer it up at dinner as "fungus".

Those who live in a modern, materially focused society are presented with many opportunities to surrender their personal power. Anytime you are exposed to the media in the form of television, movies, newspapers, magazines, you are inundated with multiple messages that tell you what you need to own, how you need to appear, how you need to smell, what hair color is sexy, what kind of beer you should drink and so forth. Implicit in all of these messages is that life would be just so much better if you did what the messages suggest. After all, for advertising to work, you need to accept the unspoken part of the message that implies that you are somehow incomplete, deficient or otherwise in need of improvement, and the use, purchase or wearing of their product will make you complete. The many smiling faces in the ad imply that you will also be happy. The object of advertising is presented as a symbol of that completeness, whether it is happiness, fame, attention, wealth, power or sex appeal.

Fashion is another symbol that has the power to control. If you have adopted and internalized a belief that fashion is important in your life and that you need to dress and live within the definition of what is "in fashion", then you will spend time, money and attention to follow what that fashion currently is. Since what is "in" and what is "out" mysteriously changes from time to time, the pursuit of living "in fashion" will require ongoing attention to fashion makers in order to keep up with the latest changes. The process of keeping up may require additional time shopping for what is currently the new fashion coupled with the expense of acquiring it. Being trendy has a cost in time, attention and money. The more important fashion is to you, the more it will control a portion of your energies. Fashion is not a "thing". It is a concept that for most people is created and defined by people they do not personally know. In the eyes of the beholder, fashion may represent any number of other symbols, such as being successful, affluent, trendy, "in" or cool. How you need to view yourself is even more important. Do you *need* to see yourself as trendy, a sharp dresser, affluent, up on fashion, cool or hot? Why? Why are those attributes so important?

The more one feels a need to embrace such a symbol, the more that symbol will hold power over you. By vesting importance and significance in a symbol such as the one called "fashion", that symbol gains power over us. The more symbols there are into which we infuse our power, the less power we retain to be who we were meant to be. Thus, the very symbols we created become our master, and we become their servant. We do this more than we know.

The point of this discussion is to step back and look at some common items from another perspective as an exercise in recalibrating our perceptions. The same analogy can easily be applied to conventional medicine. Notice that when we change our perspective, we may change how we feel and how we relate to something. Doing so can play an important part in how we view our own health, the issue of disease, the power of the diagnosis and our personal power to recover and overcome. The word-symbol we call a "diagnosis" can convey a powerful emotional message, and, sometimes, a death sentence along with it. Hearing the diagnosis of "cancer" can elicit a powerful emotional and psychological response. But how much different would the emotional response be if the physician said, "The tests indicate that you have a localized area of unregulated cell division?" While the words mean the same thing, they convey two different impacts.

A diagnosis is a symbol. It is a name or term created by men and women in medicine to describe some pathology, pathological process or group of symptoms. Being a name, it describes something else. It is not a thing anymore than you are your name. But as with fashion, we can start chasing the symbol and lose sight of that which the symbol was created to represent. In such instances, we may start looking for what makes the arthritis supposedly go away rather than looking for what is driving joint inflammation. Or, we may look for a drug to lower a laboratory value, such as cholesterol, without necessarily changing our risk. The difference between the two perspectives is vital.

If we have adopted, consciously or unconsciously, the belief that the physician knows best about our bodies and our health, then we give that physician extraordinary credit and power in our health decisions. If our definition of "physician" is defined to be *only* those who hold the MD credential and practice so-called "regular medicine", then we may exclude other healers from our experience based on our beliefs about who is a "real doctor" and who is not. This exclusion is how other medical modalities became excluded from the field of medicine. The homeopath, the osteopath, the chiropractor, the herbalist, the acupuncturist, the nutritionist and others were "defined out" by those who held legal and financial power. During my 30-plus years in practice, I have been frequently amazed by how many ostensibly educated people would dismiss a specific health or treatment modality by saying they did not believe in it. Such a person might say, "I don't believe in homeopathy" or "I don't believe in nutrition", even when they knew nothing about the subject! Somewhere, they had accepted the belief that a particular approach to health was either not a legitimate health practice or not right for them. So, here is the million-dollar question: What if the answer to your health issue was to be found in one of the therapies you "don't believe in" or haven't heard of yet? What if your decision to exclude one therapy or another is a primary reason why you are still looking for help? What if you discover a therapeutic approach, an herb or a treatment that is not accessible to you in the country in which you live? Are we willing to sentence ourselves to continued suffering due to our shortsightedness or simplistic beliefs?

Medical staff in hospitals may refer to the elderly widow who is hospitalized for acute gastrointestinal distress as "the gallbladder in Room 304". I have seen clients construct their entire lives around their illness or syndrome to such a point that without the illness they would not know what to do with their lives or how to interact with others. I remember a woman in her early 40s who had been recently been diagnosed with multiple sclerosis (MS). She was extremely busy redesigning her new house with wider doorways, wider hallways, a ramp to the front door and all of the other physical structures that would make life more comfortable when she was finally wheelchair bound. She came to see me for an initial consultation at the urging of a good friend and neighbor who believed that nutrition might help her to in some way slow down the advance of the MS or maybe even reverse its progression. When I met with this woman, we spoke of the many possibilities that she could explore to see if she could help modulate her immune system's attack on her body. She listened politely but chose not to pursue anything suggested. She was, after all, busy with her new house design and the inevitability of her disability. Her doctor had told her, "There is nothing you can do", which she evidently took to heart as true and thus lived out her belief.

Illness can provide a patient with a power over others that they might not ordinarily possess without their condition. For example, declining an invitation to a boring afternoon luncheon with your least favorite Aunt Betty is far easier to accomplish if one opts out due to a migraine. Few people will blame a person for having a migraine. After all, we don't have control over migraines. Or do we?

In the early 1980s, I attended a seminar with Dr. Bernard Siegel, a popular physician who was pioneering the concept of mind-body medicine. His message was radical talk for those early years. In that day-long seminar, Dr. Siegel made many statements that I found very difficult to accept, one being that only about five percent of cancer patients really want to get well. How could that be? Of course, anyone with cancer would want to get well, right? If you asked those cancer patients if they wanted to get well, they would certainly say, "Yes!" But, as Dr. Siegel pointed out, only a small minority of patients would actually change their lives, habits, eating choices or thoughts in order to put that wish into action. Wishing for health is not a plan. O. Carl Simonton, MD was the other physician making waves in the conventional thinking of the time, speaking of using the mind to augment the immune response against cancer cells. This concept was the early practice of envisioning one's white blood cells mimicking Pac-Man to engulf and destroy cancer cells. Dr. Siegel and Dr. Simonton both had near miraculous success with a small number of patients, those who were truly willing to *do* that which was necessary to activate their innate healing potential.

Chapter 12

Conscious or Subconscious?

Most of us believe that our interaction with life occurs through the power of our conscious mind. Our information-based societies encourage and take great pride in the training of our logical and analytical conscious abilities. After all, we have degrees, certifications and credentials attesting to the development of our linear, left-brained capabilities. But the conscious mind can only process a limited amount of information each minute and each second. If fact, some research suggests that we can consciously process about eight to 12 bits of information per second, which is the reason why you hit a wall when trying to multitask too many elements. You only have to watch a new driver taking their first lessons to see the difficulty in coordinating all the tasks involved in driving through conscious control: checking the rear-view mirror, taking your foot off the brake, applying pressure to the accelerator, checking the side-view mirrors, monitoring speed, watching for approaching cars, monitoring distance to the car ahead and so forth. Driving is difficult to do from a purely conscious level. It becomes easy and what we call "second nature" when the subconscious mind is trained and takes over. The subconscious mind can process roughly 40,000 bits of information per second, much of which never reaches our conscious awareness. If you have been driving for years, then you probably recall a particular trip when you were engrossed in either some enjoyable music or perhaps an engaging audio book and arrived home safely, unable to recall just how you got there. You made all the necessary turns, took the proper exits, paid the toll on the turnpike and arrived home all while your conscious mind was listening to your book or music. Right? So, who was driving the car? Your subconscious mind was, and it did an excellent job getting you home!

Researchers in cognitive science tell us that we experience an average of approximately 60,000 thoughts each day. Of those 60,000 thoughts, approximately 80% are "negative thoughts". That means that approximately 48,000 thoughts each day are reinforcing a negative emotion or belief and include all the judgments you make about yourself and others. These thoughts include criticisms, valuations, comparisons, judgments and other thoughts such as, "I'm stupid", "Math is hard", "I'm not attractive enough", "I'll never get ahead", "It's rude to speak your mind", "Everyone in my family is overweight", "Rich people are selfish and shallow" or any of a thousand versions of the same idea. All of these thoughts reflect a belief, and our words and actions reflect our thoughts! All this negativity can be dangerous. As Jack Canfield, originator of the *Chicken Soup for the Soul* series, says: "All suffering comes from believing our negative thoughts."

Imagine you are walking down a busy sidewalk in a major city. As you walk past the building on your right, which happens to be a mental health hospital, a patient on the seventh floor flings open a window and yells, "You're a stupid, fat, ugly slob, and I hate you!" You see them addressing this harsh remark directly at you. Are you upset? Did that wound you? Probably not. Why? Most likely, you didn't invest any credibility or give any "power" to the comments of that mentally disturbed patient shouting from the window. You don't know them, nor do they know you! However, had those same comments been directed at you by someone you know and respect, someone in whom you vested some power, your emotional experience might have been devastatingly different. Same words, different impact? It was not the words that made the difference, but the meaning and power we invested in those words that created the experience we felt.

Part IV

Identity and Belief

Chapter 13

You and Your Health

Your health is, to a large extent, an extension and expression of your values, beliefs, priorities, habits and innate biology. Excluding accidents, your health at this moment is what you have practiced doing over the years: the sum total of all your past choices, eating patterns, environmental exposures, traumas, thoughts, joys, behaviors, stresses, nutritional deficiencies, toxicities and more, as they all washed over your genes. Genetics, once believed to be the preset determiner of current and future health, is now understood through the new biology of epigenetics to be far less controlling than previously thought. In fact, your genes function as the blueprints for making new proteins and hormones when called for. Just like the blueprint for constructing a new building, a blueprint is not self-activating. That is, it takes the construction crew to read and interpret the information in the blueprint and then carry out the instructions properly in order to have the resulting building turn out as the plan intended. The blueprint cannot turn itself on or off, no matter how detailed that blueprint may be or how well-intentioned the architect was in creating the blueprint. Neither can genes.

The environment in which the cell lives, which includes the totality of all chemical, hormonal, environmental, nutritional, toxicological, energetic and emotional influences, speaks to the cell and, hence, to our genes. Said differently, cells perceive the environment in which they live and do so via thousands of receptors present on the cell membrane. This cell membrane is an organ of perception. If we are living in a constant state of worry and fear, then our cells experience that message via the many stress-hormones that mediate the fight-or-flight response. Most people have heard of "fight-or-flight" even if they do not have a good understanding of what the phrase really means. The rapid and dramatic change in your physiology upon suddenly noticing flashing blue lights in your rear-view mirror while traveling on the highway is a noteworthy example of the "fight-or-flight" response: your heart jumps, your pulse quickens, your mouth gets dry and your palms become moist. Depending on your past experiences and social programming, your mind may be filled with a sudden sense of "Oh my God" or any of a dozen other expletives, none of which may help your situation. Contrast that experience with the physiology created by lying in a hammock on a comfortably warm late summer day, perhaps a Sunday afternoon, with all of your responsibilities addressed, the ever-present to-do list nicely checked off and nothing particularly concerning in your mind. Your cells also experience that message; it is a message of "rest and repair", which is the antithesis of "fight-or-flight". In fact, your cells cannot be in both states at the same time. We are binary in that way: either A or B, not A/B. So, if we understand this important concept, taking time off on Sundays, for vacations or for extended weekends is not an issue of being unproductive. We are actively and productively engaged in self-repair and self-renewal, a process of "re-creation".

Chapter 14

Identity and Health

There are few experiences in life that can galvanize our attention as intensely as illness and disease. Taken in the positive, illness can serve as a catalyst for growth and a reevaluation of our lives and priorities. Taken for the worst, illness can literally destroy us. Although it does not always seem as such, we are all offered a decision in terms of how we will deal with the situation.

Western medicine places great emphasis on identifying and naming illnesses, diseases and, now, so-called syndromes as they arise in populations. Once limited to single-cause, acute illnesses, such as tuberculosis, typhus or syphilis, where the specific illness was caused by a single, identifiable bacteria, the illnesses and infirmities common to the hurried and frenetic members of fully Westernized cultures are frequently multi-symptom and multi-system with multiple, often poorly identified, underlying causes. These illnesses include such conditions as: chronic fatigue syndrome (CFS), fibromyalgia, post-traumatic stress disorder (PTSD), persistent developmental delay (PDD) and autistic spectrum disorders (ASD), to name a few. Even more confusing is that many syndromes are often a collection of other conditions, renamed and recoded for easy identification and accounting within the economic structure of modern medicine.

The danger arises when we accept and become one with the illness. The diagnosis becomes our identity and the lens through which we see ourselves, others and the world. We give our power to the label and make ourselves powerless to overcome the condition. How do we do that? In happens in part by seeing the disease as an entity *separate* from us and then merging with it rather than seeing the disease as an expression of an imbalance or process occurring within. When people speak of their illness, you can readily see where they are in this spectrum of identity. For example, "I am depressed" is a vastly different statement than "I am experiencing feelings of depression". If you were to take a bath, you would probably say, "I am taking a bath", meaning to convey the fact that you are having the experience of bathing. You would not merge your experience of bathing with your identity and say, "I am a bath". So, are you anxious? Are you fatigued? Or, are you experiencing the feeling of anxiety? Are you currently experiencing the sensation of fatigue?

"I am disabled" is an even more powerful identity that can have devastating consequences to your sense of self, your sense of personal power and how others see you. Even if you have some specific physical, metabolic or mental deficit, more than likely there are aspects of you that are quite gifted. Have you ever met anyone who is disabled in every facet of their existence? Probably not. If someone is missing the function of sight, perhaps they are gifted in voice and song, as in the case of Andrea Bocelli. If another person's body is severely limited in physical mobility, perhaps their mind is profoundly gifted with insight or understanding, as in the case of British theoretical physicist and cosmologist Stephen Hawking, who dictates his books with the aid of modern technology due to the physical limitations arising from a motor neuron disease. We are all, in fact, differentially able. Our abilities are more of a matter of degree than anything else.

I make this point not to endorse so-called politically correct language, but rather to remove the power from the word-symbol "disabled". I think the negative impact from defining one's self as "disabled" is on par with defining yourself as a "consumer". A consumer? What a degrading image that creates! While it is true that to live in this

3-D physical world we do by necessity "consume", it is *not* who we are. Rather, we are creators, each and every one of us! Each day you create your thoughts, goals, desires, behaviors, pursuits, laughter, deeds, emotional responses and experience of life! You are the genesis of all manner of intangible thoughts and inspirations that motivate and move you. When you combine your creative forces with your will and force of action, you make the intangible become tangible. Before there could be a light bulb, someone had to first create the idea of a light bulb!

But the power of our belief in symbols goes even deeper than that. Modern medicine, with its heavy reliance on pharmaceuticals, often uses the term "placebo" disparagingly to discredit the healing that occurs due to a belief in a medicine or a treatment. The statement "Oh, it is only a placebo effect" is meant to imply that healing created by the mind and based on a *belief* in a treatment is not real and that so-called real healing can only be due to a chemical. Odd, don't you think? A good definition of placebo would be: The healing or improvement in symptoms due to the patient's belief in a treatment when that treatment has no known therapeutic benefit. Or, said differently, a treatment that is successful only because the patient believes it will be successful.

In his book *The Biology of Belief*, Dr. Bruce Lipton describes an experiment illustrating the power of the placebo effect where patients with debilitating knee pain were divided into two groups. The first group underwent real knee surgery, and the second group received a sham surgery. In the sham surgery, the surgeon made an incision in the knee and sewed it up again. Those patients believed they were receiving the corrective surgery and recovered just as well as those patients who received the real surgery. One of the patients in the placebo surgery group who walked with the aid of a cane prior to the sham surgery was able to discard his cane afterwards and even play basketball with his grandchildren! When this gentleman was informed of the nature of his surgery two years later, he remarked, "In this world anything is possible when you put your mind to it. I know that your mind can work miracles."

Wouldn't it be nice to experience true healing based on your belief in the treatment? Wouldn't doing so result in fewer side effects? Why don't we investigate the power of belief as a means to healing? Wouldn't that be safer, better and far less costly than suppressing symptoms by pharmacological means? Why is symptom suppression considered healing, anyway?

Chapter 15

Placebo's Evil Twin

Most people do not realize that there is a dark side to the placebo effect; an evil twin, so to speak, called a "nocebo". Yes, the nocebo effect is equally powerful and can cause pain, suffering, illness and even death. A nocebo can be defined as: a harmless substance that when taken by a patient results in adverse effects due to negative expectations or the psychological state of the patient. Consequently, we have the nocebo effect.

As the definition states, the harmful effects arise from the negative expectations (or *beliefs*) about the substance. A nocebo effect could arise from taking a drug or undergoing a procedure, treatment, surgery or other intervention due. The harmful effect is due to the person's belief about it, not from the treatment itself.

The power of the nocebo can be seen when a physician tells a cancer patient that he has six months to live, and the patient believes the doctor's assessment. You can also see its effects when a person says:

> "everyone in my family dies at 65 years old" and then they fulfill that belief,
> "arthritis runs in our family" and they develop arthritis, too,
> "everyone in my family is overweight" and they cannot, of course, lose weight,

and you can see nocebo working when a person looks up every side effect of their new medication and then finds they cannot tolerate the drug.

Years ago I visited a colleague in Canada who was treating a very difficult case of "allergic to everything". Every remedy he prescribed caused horrible reactions that were worse than the last remedy. When the patient returned three days later with the same complaint, I learned that my colleague had given her a sample of her own "safe" drinking water as her last remedy, to see what would happen. Yes, the drinking water she *knew* to be safe elicited horrible reactions when she *believed* it to be a remedy.

How many people continue to be ill despite multiple treatments? How many patients have gone to "everyone", even 14 different alternative practitioners, only to remain in the same place they started? The goal here is not to blame the patient. Having an illness or condition that is not known to your practitioner is certainly possible. Yet I have seen clients who have consulted with a dozen good clinicians with no success finally respond once they assumed a different perspective on their case. We cannot discount the possibility that the nocebo effect affects millions of people.

Chapter 16

Revealing Our True Beliefs

People reveal their beliefs through their words and by their behaviors. As a clinician, I have always endeavored to listen carefully to how people describe their interactions with their primary care provider. Their choice of words can reveal their sense of power or passivity in the relationship. The most telling is when a client says, "My doctor put me on amoxicillin for my sinus infection." It is not difficult to see that the patient is not taking an active role in their own care. The language is that of passivity in the doctor-patient relationship, sometimes more akin to a parent-child relationship, at best, and victim-perpetrator, at worst.

Under ideal conditions, the interaction between patient and provider would be that of two adults deciding on a course of medical treatment based on full disclosure. Although most patients do not possess a level of knowledge of medicine or biology on parity with their physician, that is really not the major stumbling block. The interaction needs to include a frank and honest discussion of the potential benefits and limitations of any treatment proposed and how the treatment may contrast with other treatment avenues or even with doing nothing! There are a whole series of questions that the informed patient should be asking of any clinician in their quest for the best treatment. The goal is to identify the treatment that is best suited to the condition and the patient and that will lead to the best clinical outcome with the least risk.

Recognizing that few of the beliefs and attitudes we hold about heath, disease and health care in general are the product of our own deliberate thinking and research, we can begin to examine more carefully what we do believe and why. More frequently than not, these conclusions are derived from a complex mixture of opinions and distorted information we receive from other people mixed with so-called facts delivered by advertising, the media and their supposed experts. Because of the vast complexity of biology and medicine, we are reminded by these self-appointed keepers of knowledge that important decisions about our health should only be undertaken with direct supervision of their approved experts and that we are far too uneducated to accept that responsibility for ourselves. If we accept this premise as fact, then we submit our future into the hands of others. As philosopher Bertrand Russell once said, "I would never die for my beliefs because I might be wrong." In medicine, that sentiment is a literal concern. As I said earlier in this book, when we choose to live through conscious choice, we are less controlled by the manipulation of our subconscious programming.

It is no secret that the medical and pharmaceutical industries are driven by illness and disease, not by wellness. This vast, complex, multitrillion-dollar industry gains no profit from you being healthy, and there is no profit from you being dead. Somewhere in the middle is where all the money is to be made. Accordingly, there is far less profit in preventing a disease than in screenings, monitoring, early detection testing, surgical or drug treatment and long-term management of symptoms. Putting the question of economics first, it is infinitely more profitable to monitor and manage a disease over a lifetime than it is to cure a disease once, assuming such a feat was even possible. So, if you are holding on to the illusion that medical researchers and the pharmaceutical industry are searching for a cure, think again. Many, if not most, of the chronic conditions and syndromes that plague Western societies are intimately related to habits, lifestyle, nutrition and stress. Unlike acute disease wherein, say, tuberculosis is caused by a single bacterium and a single drug can be employed to successfully kill it, the chronic conditions related to habit, lifestyle, nutrition and stress are multifaceted and multisystem effects too diffuse and systemic for any drug to work. That is not to say one or more drugs will not be prescribed to ameliorate some of the symptoms, but treating symptoms is a far different goal than treating underlying causes. How can a drug treat poor sleep habits, the consequences of years of unhealthy food choices, the bioaccumulation of mercury or aluminum from vaccines, or the rampant deficiencies of iron or magnesium? When are we going to take responsibility and accept that our health starts with *us*?

Accepting the perspective that in the UK, US, Canada and other countries the so-called healthcare system is in actuality a disease-care system with the entire focus shifted to chronic care *management* makes our decisions and goals easier to define. Just listen to any pharmaceutical commercial, attend any illness-specific support group or chat with your physician and you will see the "management" theme painfully evident. You will quickly learn is that treating chronic illness is all about learning to manage and live with asthma, diabetes, arthritis, chronic fatigue syndrome, fibromyalgia, Crohn's Disease, IBS, colitis, gastritis and so on. The sobering fact is that most people contribute to or actually create their conditions by what they eat and drink, through their environmental exposures to toxins and as a result of their unmanaged stress. All these factors are aggravated by their poor sleep cycles. We do these things not because we wish to be ill and suffer, but because no one ever taught us otherwise or explained the importance of true self-care.

Diabetes is a good example. Some years ago, the cost calculation for managing the diabetic patient was approximately 33 cents of every HMO dollar spent in the US. That is a *lot* of money and an alarming statistic considering that the incidence of Type-II diabetes is doubling every ten years, and the greatest prevalence is in people in their teens and twenties. A 20 year old diagnosed with Type II diabetes will have a long and difficult life monitoring and managing the condition and the various acute problems that come with poorly controlled diabetes – and all at great cost. While it is tempting to dismiss the increasing incidence of diabetes to better and earlier diagnosis, such is not the case. Diabetes is a well-known condition that is heavily dependent on the lifestyle choices of the patient. Most clinicians who deal directly with diabetic patients appreciate that there is a "diabetic mentality" that is far more difficult to treat than the physiological interaction of glucose and insulin. This attitude will sometimes carry over when people choose to explore natural and nutritional approaches to diabetes. There is no magic pill, food, herb or vitamin that will correct diabetes *and* provide a blanket of immunity under which the diabetic may eat and drink whatever they wish.

Chapter 17

The Name Game

The naming of a disease or condition is a process we call diagnosis. Indeed, the science side of medicine requires the physician or other licensed medical person to identify the correct name for the malady experienced by a patient. In this way, we relate to our infirmity through the word-symbol name of the condition. In some cases, the name is a logical, physiology-based name, such as "gastritis", meaning an inflammation of the stomach lining. In other cases, the diagnostic name has nothing to do with an actual cause or pathology, but was adopted in honor of the person who discovered it or was the first to name it. An example is "Barrett's esophagus". There are no cells called "Barrett cells", and the name is not based on a cause. Today, many diagnoses are simply the name given to a specific collection of other symptoms. Furthermore, disease names are periodically changed. Manic-depressive syndrome was renamed "Bipolar Disorder". Chronic heartburn is now GERD. New names help eliminate the stigma that may be attached to earlier names and help people accept their labels more readily. New names also allow for a new marketing campaign.

We create all sorts of word-symbols for every aspect of our lives, including word-symbols for various states of health and illness and our state of mind. Curiously, although we are the creators of these word-symbols, we frequently give them power over us. People often refer to a disease as if it was something that jumped out of the bushes and attacked them. For example, consider statements such as "He was stricken with MS", "She had a bad gall bladder attack" or "I had an attack of colitis". Laboring under the supposition that we have been attacked, we are encouraged to wage war against this thing we call the disease. We "fight" a cold. We have a "war" on cancer. We "knock the fever down". It is a model of warfare and it causes us to view the problem as distinct and separate from us.

Would we feel differently if we chose a different naming system that viewed the signs and symptoms produced as merely the particular form or pattern by which our body expressed its internal imbalances? How then might we react to a diagnosis? Could the symptom be not a "disease" but rather the natural expression of an intelligent body doing the best it can to compensate for internal imbalance or to cope with a particular challenge?

Perhaps. Consider this scenario: You are on your way home after a day-long trip to visit friends and, being hungry, you decide to stop at a local restaurant and get a chicken salad sandwich. Unbeknownst to you, the chicken salad had been left unrefrigerated too long and had spoiled. What unpleasant symptoms might your body create later that night in response to the bad chicken salad? Vomiting? Diarrhea? Both? Would you interpret this as your body being under attack? Would you assume that your body was randomly malfunctioning? No. Your body responded intelligently to eliminate the cause of the problem in the most direct and effective manner possible. While none of us would desire the experience, we can be grateful that our innate intelligence actively protected our life and health. Using an anti-diarrheal medication to suppress the natural response of diarrhea (or anti-emetic for vomiting), and thereby keeping the noxious agent in, could have more serious consequences. In almost every case you can think of, the symptoms the body creates, whether diarrhea, vomiting, sweating, erupting, fever, pain or inflammation, are the body's response to the problem, not the actual problem itself. Our thinking has been misdirected to believe that the response to the problem *is* the problem. Once we accept that premise, then finding an appropriate chemical agent to stop that function seems quite logical.

Chapter 18

Growth or Sour Grapes

Whether we understand it or not, our lives are an evolution of growth and change. When we are young, we grow in physical size, neurological complexity, language and communication skills, eye-hand coordination and countless other ways. As we reach maturity, our physical growth may slow while our need for growth transfers to other areas, such as acquiring skills, creative thinking, problem solving, spiritual understanding, personal fulfillment, relationships and those abilities and attributes that constitute "life, liberty and the pursuit of happiness." Without growth, we die, physically or spiritually. Creativity is our life force, and all humans need to exercise that creative energy in order to be fully alive.

One question that I typically ask clients who are experiencing depression is, "What do you do in your daily life that is purely creative? How do you express your creative powers?" Not surprisingly, most have *no* creative outlet or activity in their lives. Conversely, the people who seem to have a real zest for life have many creative interests, hobbies or pursuits. For many, their work is also a creative outlet. Although you could argue which came first, the zest for life or the creative interests, most depressed people feel better when they find something that allows for their creative energy to be unleashed. Perhaps this is why some philosophies regard compassion for others and for self, as an antidote to depression.

Growth and change are two sides of the same coin. Most people prefer what is known and familiar rather than that which is new and unknown, and the prospect of change can make us feel very uncomfortable. It can be downright scary. Change may be prompted by crisis or exposure to new information. The heart bypass surgical patient may be suddenly faced with the need to change long-standing eating or smoking behaviors when facing their own mortality. For people facing less urgent decision points, the need to change may appear less imperative.

Chapter 19

When it Hurts to Change

It is my observation that there are three major psychological states or perspectives that silently and almost imperceptibly keep people stuck in distress, disease, limitation and lack. Individually and collectively, these perspectives impose the greatest disability and disempower people throughout the world, but probably nowhere more so than in the US. These three states arise from a complex combination of perceptions and unspoken beliefs. In fact, they might more accurately be called "memes". The Oxford English Dictionary defines a meme as "an element of a culture or system of behaviour passed from one individual to another by imitation or other non-genetic means." Whether we can accurately define them as "memes", The System (which we will discuss in an upcoming section) creates and reinforces these psychological conditions.

What are they? Simply stated, they are:
1) **cognitive dissonance**
2) **learned helplessness**, and
3) **Stockholm Syndrome**

We will look at each of these states individually in the pages ahead to better understand how they may affect not only our thinking, but also our actions, choices and ultimately our mental and physical health.

Cognitive dissonance is probably one of the most pervasive and powerful forces operating today. In fact, I believe it is one of the biggest factors that keep this world and its people locked in behaviors leading to chronic illness, pain and poor quality of life. The term simply comes from the two words: "cognitive", meaning awareness or knowledge, and "dissonance", meaning discomfort or inner stress. When our existing belief system is confronted with new information, ideas, values or emotional experiences that challenge the beliefs we already hold, we tend to experience a level of discomfort called "dissonance". Most commonly, this dissonance is created when a belief is *contradicted* by the new experience or new information. That inner distress may express itself through uncomfortable feelings, which may include dread, fear, anxiety, anger, surprise or embarrassment. When we experience cognitive dissonance, we can respond in one of two ways: 1) we can evaluate the new information and modify our existing map of the world accordingly, or 2) defend our map of the world and reject the new information.

To illustrate this point, let's take the case of acupuncture. Acupuncture came to the US in the 1970s and gradually gained favor in the natural health care and back to nature movements of the late 1960s. Acupuncture had been in use since 3000 BC in China and Japan and had been used for major and minor health issues along with medicinal herbs and lifestyle and dietary modification. Acupuncture had even been used as anesthesia for major surgery; yet it was not uncommon for many Americans, especially physicians and people trained in western science, to say, "I don't believe in acupuncture". US medical doctors held the academic opinion that acupuncture was "unproven". So, let's put that into perspective. Acupuncture, a technique that had been in continuous use to treat millions of people for centuries on more than one continent, was "unproven", while the use of small doses of highly toxic chemicals to suppress the body's expression of specific symptoms or groups of symptoms and utilized only over a period of 70 years was "established" and "scientific"? Today, the established death rate from pharmaceuticals properly prescribed by licensed and trained physicians makes prescription drugs the third leading cause of death in the US. If you add up all the deaths caused by modern medicine, it is by several accounts the leading cause of death in America. But most people will accept modern medicine and its outcomes as "scientific" and "proven". Without the proper perspective, we let ourselves be fooled. As so succinctly stated by Soren Kierkegaard: "There are two ways to be fooled: One is to believe what isn't so; the other is to refuse to believe what is so."

Our natural aversion to pain and discomfort prompts a strong desire to reduce this internal unease quickly to restore internal harmony, so most people will react by quickly rejecting, refuting or misperceiving the information without the benefit of further research or investigation. If people really feel threatened, they may recruit support from family or friends who share their same original point of view in an effort to build a consensus that will bolster against any feeling of vulnerability. The thinking goes, "Of course, if we all agree, then it must be true!" German sociologist and psychoanalyst Erich Fromm makes the point clearly in stating: "The fact that millions of people share the same vices does not make these vices virtues, the fact that they share so many errors does not make the errors to be truths, and the fact that millions of people share the same form of mental pathology does not make these people sane". In some cases, not only are the facts refuted or rejected, but also the messenger may need to be thoroughly degraded and discredited in an effort to eradicate any appearance that the challenging information is valid. Hence the adage, "Don't shoot the messenger".

Take a moment and rewind back to a point in time when you felt that internal discomfort, the unease created by a potential threat to your beliefs. That feeling is, in disguise, the signal that growth and change may be at your doorstep. Yes, both an opportunity and a choice are presented by discomfort. Feeling uneasy when presented with new information is analogous to feeling hunger when your body wants to signal it is time to eat or yawning when your body is tired. You were just never told of the connection. Updating our map of the world is important as we progress through life, and there are consequences for not doing so. Just as you might get lost traveling to a new destination using an out-of-date GPS database, your map of the world cannot direct you to the destination you desire if it does not match reality. Every time we deny ourselves the opportunity to grow, we expand the gap between our map and reality. And like a rubber band being stretched too far, at some point, during something we call "crisis", the band will snap back. The key, then, is to redefine what that the discomfort arising from cognitive dissonance really means.

So, just how do we deal with this internal discomfort? The response of denial can be made in one of three ways. In **simple denial**, we deny the reality or truthfulness of the unpleasant fact altogether. We might say something like, "No, I don't believe that aspartame is bad for you" or "No, they wouldn't put fluoride in the water if it was bad for you." Although people make such statements, they have rarely invested any time researching the topic through independent sources to check out the facts. Adopting a myth that eases our distress is easier than working toward a truthful understanding.

In a form of denial called **minimization**, we admit the fact but then deny how serious it is. For example, we might say "Yeah, I heard about bisphenol A, but I don't think it's that bad for you" or "Well, there is only a little bit of mercury in that vaccine". Again, how seriously an issue is allowed to affect us also depends on our level of understanding about it. Did this person do any homework or research to support their conclusion about the harmfulness of BPA? Probably not. Is 300 nanograms of mercury in a vaccination a "little bit" when far less can cause neurological inflammation? Such statements are more than likely self-soothing delusions intended to restore a person's internal comfort and allow them to avoid dealing with it.

In the third form of denial, often called **projection**, we may admit both the fact and seriousness but deny any responsibility in the situation. Common examples of projection statements are, "Well, I'm not going to give up my cell phone! I have to use it for work", or "I know GMOs are really bad, but I don't have time to read all the labels on the products that I buy in the grocery store". In this response, we abdicate responsibility, negate our personal power and blame an external factor for the consequences. But whether we want to point fingers and attach blame to others does not change the risk attached to eating GMO foods. This attitude is a march toward full self-victimization.

The unfortunate fact is: Denial kills. The diabetic who is unwilling or unable to accept the seriousness of their condition may lose toes, feet and legs to gangrene on their way to losing their life. The Crohn's patient who will not address the level of stress in their life or their gluten intolerance may end up with a colostomy and all of the difficulties that go with it. The arthritis patient who will swallow all sorts of noxious immuno-suppressive drugs but cannot swallow the fact that they are holding onto tremendous levels of anger and resentment will deal with years of pain and limitation. The migraine patient who would rather have episodes of debilitating pain than omit the dairy or wheat that is driving the condition uses the principle of cause and effect against themselves. How many more conditions can we name? What will it take to snap us into reality? Is suffering really the only message that we will hear?

For thirty years, I had a small 4" x 5" hand-made sign on my desk. The words were simple: "Self-discipline is not as great an inconvenience as Disease is." For while the discomfort generated by cognitive dissonance is quite real, I would submit that the discomfort generated by embracing denial is ultimately greater. As Ayn Rand so aptly stated, "You can avoid reality, but you cannot avoid the consequences of avoiding reality."

The interplay between cognitive dissonance and denial are beautifully illustrated in the concept of sour grapes. What do sour grapes have to do with our thinking processes? The phrase "sour grapes" refers to the classic fable *The Fox and the Grapes* by Aesop (ca. 620–564 BC). In this story, a fox sees some high-hanging grapes that he wishes to eat. Though he is creative, the fox is unable to devise a way to reach the grapes and so he decides that the grapes are probably not worth eating anyway. To make himself feel better, the fox creates the justification that the grapes are probably not ripe and are, in fact, probably quite sour. Hence, the term "sour grapes". This example follows a clear and oft-repeated pattern: We desire something, find it unattainable and reduce our internal dissonance by criticizing it.

How can you tell when you or someone around you is in cognitive distress? You can usually tell by their response to new information, new experiences or new behaviors that conflict with their internal map. Attempts to silence or dismiss the challenging information can be seen in how people respond:

- "You're crazy, I just can't believe that is true!"
- "Oh well, we're all gonna die of something anyway."
- "My motto is: Everything in moderation."
- "Boy, he's really 'out there', isn't he?"
- "That's being negative!"
- "I didn't want it anyway."
- "That's just some crazy conspiracy theory."
- "Can we talk about something pleasant?"
- "I just can't deal with that right now."
- "Where did you get that information, from some crazy Internet site?"

The desire to restore our internal comfort is a powerful force and one that operates silently in the background nearly 100% of the time, even if we have to lie to ourselves to feel better. We are hardwired to be attracted to pleasure and averse to pain. To help accomplish this goal, we create many self-soothing delusions about food and health so we can avoid change.

If you listen to any of the voices emanating from old network television or print media (traditionally called mainstream media), you will notice how insane much of what you see and hear really is: Silly stories, gossip, drama with no meaning, crazy people doing stupid things and an emphasis on entertainment and fabricated controversies. The heroic recovery of a cat that fell down a well in a small village you never heard of gets the same airtime as the latest war, bank failures or government cover-up. Or a winter storm arrives in an area that normally gets winter storms, and reporters are asking people standing out in the snow what they think about the snow! This is news?

What you will find, if you look closely, is that the important stories are not even covered. The Media appears to offer you everything and anything to keep your mind distracted in order to divert your awareness away from more relevant issues. Simultaneously, however, it is drowning out the softer inner voice of the *true you*. You have to be still enough and quiet enough to allow space for that voice of spirit and intuition to be heard. Media and society feeds you a nearly constant stream of information that keeps you in a state of cognitive dissonance. You may watch a television news story about the latest SWAT raid that seized a couple of kilos of marijuana at a local house followed three minutes later by a story about a ten-year-old girl in grade school arrested under the so-called zero-tolerance drug policy adopted by the school board for having an unauthorized cough drop in her pocket. Meanwhile, throughout the entire 30-minute news program, all you see is commercial after commercial for the latest cholesterol drug, asthma inhaler, anti-inflammatory drug or SSRI. What does the mind do with such conflicting statements? Drugs are bad? Drugs are good? It does not make sense until you understand that the dollars involved in the so-called war on drugs pales in comparison to the dollars involved in promoting governmentally approved drugs.

Also on the news, you might hear a story that some European country is in such debt that they cannot pay their bills; they are cutting back police, teachers and other essential services. Yet, two minutes later in the same story, they will assert that the solution is for them to borrow more money to keep going. Or a story about high unemployment numbers quickly followed by another story of police shutting down a children's lemonade stand because they didn't have the right permit. Or that the FDA is conducting SWAT team raids on raw milk coops and Amish farmers who dare to sell their cheese to their neighbors. The insanity and inherent contradictions of all of this input creates a chronic state of internal distress and dissonance, which primes you to react emotionally in other areas of your life. Is it any wonder that Americans consume 80% of the painkillers produced in the world today?

The term **learned helplessness** arises from within psychiatry and psychology circles. It is defined in the Oxford English Dictionary as "a condition in which a person suffers from a sense of powerlessness, arising from a traumatic event or persistent failure to succeed." Some professionals believe it may be an underlying cause of depression. An example of learned helplessness is a person who feels the need to rely on others to do almost everything. There are people who will go to the emergency room to treat a cold or run to the physician with every sniffle or sneeze rather than learn how to take proper care of themselves. Perhaps the experience of a viral infection creates a feeling of helplessness. If they witness an injury, they don't jump in to help, but instead call 911 and then standby and wait. Any sense of helplessness may be reinforced by the fear of being sued for their helpfulness. If they have issues with the neighbor, they will call the police to handle it for them. If there is a bear or other unexpected wildlife in the backyard, they call the authorities. (I don't know about you, but when I was growing up the good people that worked as police and firefighters were "public servants", not "authorities.") The important point is that the personal senses of self-care, responsibility, personal strength and self-reliance have been largely erased.

If you look up a disease in most current medical books or on a good medical web site, you can learn a lot about how the disease is diagnosed, what lab tests are usually ordered, which drugs are most appropriate and what the complications could be if the problem is not successfully treated. But what you rarely find is clear information about the *cause*. Yes, that pesky little thing called "the cause." Saying that arthritis is an inflammation of the joints so the cause of the inflammation is arthritis is not sufficient. The real question is: what is the cause of the inflammation? What's the cause of diabetes? What's the cause of bipolar disorder? Yet, these unanswered questions do not seem to slow the medical system down from offering treatments for conditions for which they admit they do not understand the cause. Many newer illnesses are called "syndromes" and are even more poorly understood, such as fibromyalgia, Chronic Fatigue Syndrome, chronic Lyme disease and others that may leave the dependent patient either feeling that their condition is incurable or, worse, waiting for a new drug or vaccine to come along and rescue them.

Chapter 20

A Few Words About "The System"

Let me emphasize that the overall story here is a decidedly positive one with, I believe, a happy outcome. But for a few minutes, let's talk a little more about The System that I have alluded to so we can better understand how it affects you, your life, your health and your decisions. Only by understanding what The System is, how it operates, what its objectives are and how we gave it our power can we hope to reclaim our personal power.

As we discussed earlier, the societies in which we all live are comprised of various systems and subsystems that serve important functions. The educational, legal, medical, banking and financial systems are some of the systems that we interact with and rely upon in a complex, functioning society. Since these systems are by necessity all interlocked and interconnected, society itself has become a system of systems. Government is also a system; in many countries, it is thoroughly woven into the fabric of society. At this point in the 21st Century, most governments have become authoritarian in nature to one degree or another. Even those that were ostensibly established to serve the will of its people have changed in significant ways. The very nature of government is to work toward increasing its power; because there is never enough power from the government's perspective, all governments seek to become totalitarian (that is, to acquire total power). No matter what form of government we examine—oligarchy, monarchy, plutocracy, democracy or republic—those in government seek to expand the power and reach of government. Honestly, can you think of one government around the world today that places service to its citizens above the desire to control? For every new power gained by government, a power is taken from the people. Governing is, as they say, a zero-sum game.

Today, societies and their governments are largely the product of powerful special interests that pull strings from the shadows. This fact is no longer a controversial concept nor is it a secret, and many have spoken about it from the outside and the inside, which will be discussed later. Slowly, over decades, these powerful interests have structured the education system, the financial system, the media, the medical system, the legal system and government to their own designs. Indeed, modern society has become an inter-locking system of systems that has its own interests at heart. It is most unabashedly evident in medicine, in media and in the institutions we call government. While exploring the nature of this system in any great detail is not in the scope of this book, it is important that we acknowledge its existence as a force with which we interact, knowingly or not. For the sake of simplicity, I shall refer to these systems within society as "The System", and you can make your own judgments about it as you prefer. The medical industry is just one subsystem within the overall System, and it emulates the same goals and principles.

I think the character Morpheus in the first movie **The Matrix** had it right when he was explaining to Neo that the Matrix was "the world that has been pulled over your eyes to blind you from the truth". Morpheus goes on to say that Neo, like everyone else, was born into bondage…. "born into a prison that you cannot smell or taste or touch….. A prison for your mind". Later, Morpheus explains that most of those people were not ready for true freedom and because of their hopeless dependence on that system, they would fight to protect it.

Well, that's a movie. Is there really a System? Is there any objective evidence that those who think of themselves as the governing elite and pull the strings of power have vastly different goals and interests than you do? How you wish to characterize this System, I shall leave up to you. Whether you choose to label it as "good" or "evil", "conspiracy" or "coincidence" is really immaterial to the points that follow. (Caution: cognitive dissonance may be engaging now!) To help answer this question, we will examine a limited number of selected quotes from notable and connected people. For those readers who wish to review a more extensive list along with important background information, please visit the website: www.thrivemovement.com. Additional quotations are also posted at www.mindmythsbook.com.

In 1953, Bertrand Russell wrote in his book *The Impact of Science on Society*:

> Diet, injections, and injunctions will combine, from a very early age, to produce the sort of character and the sort of beliefs that the authorities consider desirable, and any serious criticism of the powers that be will become psychologically impossible. Even if all are miserable, all will believe themselves happy, because the government will tell them that they are so.

In the same book, Russell goes on to say that really "high-minded people" were indifferent to the suffering of other people and that the most effective ways of creating a stable population was through the use of birth control, "infanticide or really destructive wars" and the creation of a general level of misery "except for a powerful minority".

In 1962, Julian Huxley spoke enthusiastically about an entirely new class of central nervous system drugs that could "energize" people's mental processes without doing any obvious harm. But the most revealing insight comes from a later statement about how these new drugs could be used: "In the hands of a dictator these substances in one kind or the other could be used with, first of all, complete harmlessness, and the result would be, you can imagine a euphoric that would make people thoroughly happy even in the most abominable circumstances".

In a 1962 Berkeley speech, Aldous Huxley spoke enthusiastically about how emerging technologies could be used to keep people subdued.

> That we are in the process of developing a whole series of techniques which will enable the controlling oligarchy who have always existed and presumably will always exist, to get people to love their servitude.

Zbigniew Brzezinski, advisor to President Barrack Obama (United States) and to numerous previous US Presidents, had this to say in his book, *Between Two Ages: America's Role in the Technetronic Era*:

> The technetronic era involves the gradual appearance of a more controlled society. Such a society would be dominated by an elite, unrestrained by traditional values. Soon it will be possible to assert almost continuous surveillance over every citizen and maintain up-to-date complete files containing even the most personal information about the citizen.

Brezesinski also points out that while the lethality of power held by government is at its greatest, their power to control the "politically awakened masses" around the world was concurrently at its historical lowest level. In contrast to earlier times in history, he states: "Today it is infinitely easier to kill a million people than to control a million people".

In his book *Memoirs*, David Rockefeller discusses the long history of political extremists at both ends of the political spectrum attacking his family for their tremendous influence over American economic and political institutions. But Rockefeller also reveals his real agenda in this statement:

> Some even believe we are part of a secret cabal working against the best interests of the United States, characterizing my family and me as 'internationalists' and of conspiring with others around the world to build a more integrated global political and economic structure--one world, if you will. If that's the charge, I stand guilty, and I am proud of it.

Woodrow Wilson (28th President of the United States) spoke of his understanding the hidden power structure in his 1913 book The New Freedom when he said:

> Since I entered politics, I have chiefly had men's views confided to me privately. Some of the biggest men in the United States, in the field of commerce and manufacture, are afraid of something. They know that there is a power somewhere so organized, so subtle, so watchful, so interlocked, so complete, so pervasive, that they better not speak above their breath when they speak in condemnation of it.

Joseph Kennedy, the father of John F. Kennedy and Robert F. Kennedy and who served as United States Ambassador, echoed Wilson's sentiments in stating: "Fifty men have run America, and that's a high figure". Whether we go forward in time or back in time, we find key government figures revealing the same experiences. In 1952, US Supreme Court Justice Felix Frankfurter said: "The real rulers in Washington are invisible, and exercise power from behind the scenes." In 1933, Franklin Roosevelt (32nd President of the United States) traced this theme back to even an earlier point in US history in stating:

"The real truth of the matter is, as you and I know, that a financial element in the larger centers has owned the government since the days of Andrew Jackson." In 1906, Theodore "Teddy" Roosevelt (26th President of the United States) expressed a less approving toward this hidden power in his statement:

> Behind the ostensible government sits enthroned an invisible government owing NO allegiance and acknowledging NO responsibility to the people. To destroy this invisible government, to befoul this unholy alliance between corrupt business and corrupt politics is the first task of the statesmanship of today.

In 1917, U.S. Congressman Oscar Callaway addressed his concern regarding the control of the press by the super wealthy as recorded in the US Congressional Record on February 9, 1917. Callaway spoke of how the J.P. Morgan interests gathered 12 key men from within the newspaper industry in the US and how they, in turn, selected the key newspapers from around the country. Callaway stated: "These 12 men worked the problems out by selecting 179 newspapers, and then began, by an elimination process, to retain only those necessary for the purpose of controlling the general policy of the daily press throughout the country." He went on to say that with the purchase of only 25 key newspapers, they would be successful in "the suppression of everything in opposition to the wishes of the interests served."

And lastly, we have this somewhat famous dictum from Dr. Joseph Paul Goebbels, Reich Minister for Propaganda, 1933-1945, Nazi Germany:

> The lie can be maintained only for such time as the State can shield the people from the political, economic and/ or military consequences of the lie. It thus becomes vitally

important for the State to use all of its powers to repress dissent, for the truth is the mortal enemy of the lie, and thus by extension, the truth is the greatest enemy of the State.

These excerpts are just a tiny sampling of the innumerable quotations, articles, books and references that support the idea that the systems within society operate on a far different level than appearances would suggest. (I have provided additional quotations on the website: www.mindmythsbook.com for those who wish to increase the depth of their understanding.) Interestingly, no effort has been made to hide any of this evidence. Those who control the System rely upon the cognitive dissonance built into the System (and our minds) to dissuade most people from ever considering that such a coordinated construct could even exist. This System, as expressed through the subordinate medical system, is the invisible force you push up against when you want to treat your cancer with so-called alternative methods, when you want to drink farm-fresh raw milk, when you decline vaccinations for yourself or for your child or when you demand clear labeling laws for GMO foods. If you live in the US or in several other countries, you are effectively held hostage to rules, laws and regulations that are enforced against your free will and conscience under the guise of protecting you. Ostensibly, we all need protection from ourselves! However, despite the advance of such regulatory limitations on our lives, we can paradoxically identify evidence of Stockholm Syndrome, primarily in those who have not yet begun to awaken and especially in those whose lives depend heavily on this System. If we look at a definition for **Stockholm Syndrome**, we find it is: "an emotional attachment to a captor formed by a hostage as a result of continuous stress, dependence, and a need to cooperate for survival". – Dictionary.com

Your medical insurance policy will cover only those medical services, treatments and prescriptions approved by the physicians they hired to sit on their claims review board. Without the financial means to go outside the medical system and self-pay, you are certainly held captive by the medical industry. The System makes huge profits from medical services and is at the same time heavily invested in the junk-food industry and the promotion of the very foods that contribute to chronic illness.

Financial coverage for the $80,000 coronary bypass surgery combined with the cost for nearly endless monthly supplies of supposedly life-saving medications that claim to manage the symptoms of heart disease can be a powerful bonding force, creating a captor and hostage relationship in those who are susceptible. Some may still go as far as to exclaim the wishful sentiment that "the US has the best medical care in the world!" The facts would easily challenge the veracity of that statement, which is founded in emotion, wishful thinking and dependence.

When we take a closer look at how The System operates, we find that it has an active, built-in bias that encourages and discourages certain behaviors and thought processes. Quietly, underneath the banner of "helping", The System works to:

- encourage dependence;
- diminish self-reliance; and
- keep you locked in to a left brain–dominant view of reality disconnected from nature and your intuition.

In order to flourish, The System *needs* you to believe in several key myths:

- that you are merely a mind and a body;
- that you are a *name*;
- that the five-sense, what-you-see-is-what-you-get reality is all there is;
- that quiet, reflective time is unproductive;

- that most of your non-work time should be directed toward "fun";
- that acquiring material stuff is the primary goal and the real measure of success;
- that acquiring stuff will lead to your personal happiness;
- that being in debt is both normal and good;
- that you need the System to protect you;
- that leaving the System would be catastrophic and lead to your impoverishment; and
- that the System is always serving your best interests.

It may be helpful to interject here that myths are very much like narcotics. Believing them distorts our perception of reality and alters how we think. Myths that make us feel better are frequently addictive. You believe 100% in what you believe, and, because humans are all basically pleasure attracted and pain averse, we tend to hold on to those myths and beliefs because we want to feel good (or at the very least less uncomfortable than with another perspective).

You can see these principles in operation everywhere. If you have any sustained interaction with modern medicine, then you will observe that it has its own set of rules that members largely adhere to. These rules include:

Rule #1: Maintain the system
Rule #2: Maintain control over the patient
Rule #3: Encourage dependence
Rule #4: Discourage and discredit any competing medical models
Rule #5: Use the power of the State to protect your interests

You can see this at work quite readily. Modern medicine prescribes drugs to manage symptoms rather than resolve the condition;

insurance co-payments work to obscure the real cost of the drugs and to make the therapeutic playing field both uneven and uncompetitive. How costly would the nutrients, herbs, homeopathic remedies or treatments by your acupuncturist be compared to the drugs *if you had to pay the full cost?*

Years ago I worked with a mother whose 24-month-old child had just finished her 24th antibiotic prescription for "ear infections". At this stage of her daughter's young life, Mom was now becoming concerned that something was not right. Although she had to drive many hours to visit me at my office, she was committed to finding a better way. We spoke about the possibility that her daughter might be sensitive to dairy products, which were a large part of the family's diet. I suggested that she eliminate all dairy products from her diet and that, when the next ear infection occurred, we might be able to break the cycle by actively supporting the child's immune system to get through the infection. I knew that there would be another ear infection and so prepared Mom for that eventuality. Had I not done so, she could have mistakenly concluded, "Nothing is working". When the next ear infection occurred, we spoke about what measures she could do for her daughter to support her through the experience. (Not being a physician, I am not trained or licensed to perform physical exams on clients, so I always recommend that parents seek a medical evaluation whenever they have doubts.)

It is important to note that Dad was not happy that Mom was seeing what he thought of as a "quack" (me), and so they visited the pediatrician for a diagnosis with that next inevitable ear infection. Not surprisingly, the pediatrician prescribed another antibiotic (the 25th). Mom decided to share what she was attempting to do to break the cycle. Unfortunately, the pediatrician was not only unsupportive, but also outraged that she even considered not giving her daughter yet another prescription. In fact, he was so vehement about the matter that he told Mom that he was going to call the pharmacy to make sure she filled the prescription and that if she did not, he was going to call Child Protective Services to come take her daughter for "medical neglect". This sad-but-true story had a happy ending. Mom filled the prescription but did not use it. She followed my suggestions, and her daughter came through quite nicely. And that was the last ear infection she ever had! Even Dad became a believer! I relay this story because it demonstrates all of the Rules of Modern Medicine, starting with Rule #1: Maintain the system right through Rule #5: use the State to enforce your interests.

Dr. Robert Mendelsohn, pediatrician, author and professor of medicine, said for many years that pediatrics could not survive as a specialty if it were not for the use of fear and ignorance employed against the patients' parents. Isn't that odd? In almost every other service or industry, the educated buyer is encouraged. Apparently, this is not so in modern medicine. If you have ever done a lot of research and then taken a long list of questions into your primary care physician for discussion, you know how difficult it can be to get the answers you need. Dr. Mendelsohn said that modern medicine functioned more like a religion where you were expected to simply believe without asking question. Fortunately, a new generation of physicians and medical professionals is emerging who will take time to listen to patients and honestly answer their questions, but this experience is still relatively uncommon.

To my thinking, true health is resilience and vitality. With the application of healthy living principles, health allows for increasing *independence* from the practitioner and reliance upon self. Thus, any healthcare modality or practitioner that fosters greater dependence should be carefully examined. A good healthcare practitioner should at all times be working to make his or her services less and less necessary by empowering the patient.

The System is also evident in the corporate workplace, in government regulations that stifle creativity and entrepreneurship, in the legal system and in banking and finance. As the character Morpheus said in the *Matrix*: "The Matrix is everywhere, it is all around us. Even now, in this very room. You can see it when you look out your window, or when you turn on your television. You can feel it when you go to work, or when go to church or when you pay your taxes". Just substitute "System" for Matrix and it is a match.

Years ago, I heard or read a statement somewhere that put things in a nutshell: "We are all involuntarily enrolled in a system that rewards committed self-destruction." (If I could remember who said this, I would like to thank them!!) If you think about this statement, I believe you will find this perspective to be accurate. However, I also believe that the statement is only true until we awaken! Consciousness changes everything! When we awaken to our true nature; when we discover and activate our latent gifts and potentials; when we begin to reclaim our power as the creators we were meant to be; we begin to withdraw our energy from the System and strengthen ourselves. Then the choice and the power will come through the emergence of our Consciousness.

The System needs you to accept and believe the myths outlined above because it cannot survive without your support and silent obedient consent. It needs you to remain unconscious and largely distracted. The System is actually somewhat fragile in that regard. To survive and grow, the System has become quite sophisticated and adept at manipulating your mind and your body. It creates, withholds, distorts and denies the facts and information that you need to create understanding and a more accurate picture of reality. What can we say about a System that feeds your mind a diet of fear and worry while at the same time working to withhold access to the nourishing elements that allow you to thrive? The body and the mind can be manipulated through pharmaceuticals, toxic chemicals, food additives, addictive substances and behaviors, vaccines, genetically modified organisms and more. The question is: do we wish to volunteer to enroll in their experiment? Did we even understand that we were volunteering in the first place?

Consciousness, however, is immune to all of deception and manipulation. Consciousness can see past the fabricated facades and through the orchestrated illusions. Consciousness can access understanding and perspective from some other source. It has the power to set us all free. Gathering facts and data takes effort and a considerable expenditure of energy. Sifting, sorting, organizing and interpreting this information into a meaningful pattern takes even more effort. Truth, however, simply reveals itself without effort, without energy and without bias. Intuition cannot be deceived by false facts and manufactured data. All we have to do is allow ourselves to hear and understand that quiet voice of inner Consciousness to find the way!

As I said at the beginning of this section, I believe this story is a positive one with a positive outcome. You cannot undo a shift to greater Consciousness. Once I say "pink elephant", you will think of pink elephants! Through the greater collective unconscious mind shared by all people, the more people who become aware, the easier it is for those who are a few steps behind. Knowing is the proper power for doing. Johann Wolfgang von Goethe provides us with the strategy when he stated: "Knowing is not enough; we must apply. Willing is not enough; we must do".

In the last section of this book, I will offer practical suggestions for how you can begin to un-plug from the System.

Chapter 21

Believe It or Not

Eating is an especially personal experience, and everyone is an expert in what they like to eat and why. When information is presented that French fries may be unhealthy or that eight cans of a cola soft drink per day may lead to diabetes, the person who likes French fries or cola will probably respond with either a denial or a defense, such as: "Well, you are going to die of something", "Oh, I don't believe it. I've been eating French fries my entire life" or "But I like soda!"

Back in the mid-1980s, I conducted a lot of nutritional seminars to help people understand how modern clinical nutrition therapeutics could help with various health problems. During that time, therapeutic nutrition was just appearing on the radar and rapidly gaining the interest of a wider population of people. PMS, arthritis, migraine and ADD were some of the topics I would address in small groups of 25–45 people, and the attendees were fascinated with the concept that natural substances could make a real difference. But no matter how I presented the material, no matter how I referenced the science for what I was saying, every so often there would be a doubter in the audience. He (it was almost invariably a male) would say something like, "Well, all this nutrition is fine for some people, but I don't believe in it." This comment always struck me as incredible. Did this attendee really think that he was exempt from the laws of human physiology and biochemistry because he didn't "believe it"?

Looking back, the doubter's comment raises some very complicated and deep questions that I did not appreciate at the time. Indeed, could I swallow three ounces of arsenic and have no ill effects if I believe that arsenic is harmless? Could I levitate from the floor if I declare that I do not believe in gravity? Conventional thinking offers a clear, rational answer to both questions, and my science education tells me what that answer is. But on another level, I hold questions and doubts. In any case, clearly my presentation challenged some deeply held beliefs in this gentleman, and he was not about to modify his map of the world any time soon.

When we feel threatened on some level, this kind of response is almost automatic, unless you train yourself to be open minded to the possibility for growth. In people with highly trained, left brain–dominant minds, the discomfort created by cognitive conflict and the rigidity of their belief system can produce an especially powerful defensive response. This type of response is very common in lawyers, physicians, engineers or any profession that required both extensive and intensive assimilation of rules and supposed facts that later had to be regurgitated on a board exam to do the very thing you just trained to do. Redirecting any of that information into the right hemisphere of the brain and introducing new ideas, approaches or inventions (such as natural methods of treating a disease that are unapproved by the medical system) are likely to elicit rebuke and reprimands from those who are keepers of the status quo. The threat of license revocation, and, with it, the loss of livelihood and profession, is the legal dog collar that not only keeps many professionals in the box, but also causes them to vehemently defend that box! Such strong defensive responses may or may not arise from sincerity. As Martin Luter King, Jr. so aptly said: "Nothing in all the world is more dangerous than sincere ignorance and conscientious stupidity".

Chapter 22

The Seven Self-Soothing Delusions

1. A good meal cancels out a poor meal

This idea supposes that eating a croissant or doughnut for breakfast and then grabbing a processed drive-through meal for lunch can somehow be magically neutralized by eating a really good dinner. A lot of people believe this idea and then feel better about themselves for not eating three totally unhealthy meals in the day when, in fact, they ate two. I cannot tell you how many people I have heard say that they ate a lot of crappy food that day and then smile and say, "But I had a good dinner!" The truth is, if you typically eat three meals per day and only one is healthy, then one-third of your food that day was health promoting and two-thirds was detrimental. Obviously, this eating regimen is not a prescription for moving forward with your health. Every meal, every forkful of food and every sip of a beverage is quite literally an exercise in applied endocrinology that signals a message to your cells. You create and direct the messages your cells receive meal by meal, drink by drink, day by day, for the good or for the bad. Adding +1 to -2 does not equal 3.

2. Everything in moderation

This myth is so widely accepted that it can be difficult to get people to hear otherwise. It generates a whole range of thoughts and behaviors that seem justified by the myth. In many ways, this myth helps us avoid the sense of discomfort that arises from the underlying belief that eating a truly healthy diet is a matter of constant deprivation and sacrifice. Somehow, we have been conditioned to accept the belief that eating foods that are unhealthy is fun and enjoyable and healthy foods are unappealing. Yes, processed foods often do taste quite good. Food scientists chemically engineer them to do so. Yes, they may be linked to pleasant memories or experiences from earlier in life, such as when your grandmother came to visit and brought pies and cookies. Or perhaps, those special foods were used as treats to reward the "good girl" and "good boy" for accomplishments or "proper" behaviors.

The myth of moderation is based on a collection of underlying, poorly defined ideas and beliefs. Some of the many problems with this myth are:

1) no one agrees on the definition of moderation;
2) it is both the frequency of ingestion and the amount ingested that affects us;
3) what one person tolerates another may not;
4) we are each genetically predisposed to express different conditions and diseases depending on the messages that our food delivers; and, lastly,
5) there are some things that are simply unhealthy at any level of exposure, even if eaten infrequently or in small amounts, such as rancid fat, organophosphate pesticides, Bisphenol A, mercury, etc.

But people are people, and they always want to know how much and how often they can eat unhealthy foods and not see anything bad happen. They want to know how they can get away with it. It is a fair question that is frequently asked.

The answer is rarely forthcoming in black-and-white clarity. Silent, internal physiological reactions are not always revealed by obvious external signs of symptoms. From a sensory perspective, most of us are not equipped to sensitively and accurately gauge how we are doing internally. Further, genetic predisposition, past nutritional history, past medical history, past trauma, and past environmental exposures are all factors that affect how much your body will tolerate, with the latter always changing.

But there may be an answer. In most cultures, special days are honored during the year as "feast days", usually to commemorate certain events, such as religious or spiritual observances. We call them "holidays", and during such observations it is common to partake of special foods or drink as part of the celebration. Each culture has its traditions and favorites. And what kind of celebration would it be without the special sweets and treats that everyone looks forward to?

If our day-to-day diet was founded on healthy, whole and fresh foods, I have no doubt that the impact of "holiday eating" would be minimal. Part of being healthy is having resilience, and any healthy man or woman should tolerate and enjoy the special foods consumed infrequently on these holidays. Some might argue that the social and emotional benefits far outweigh the physiological effects of the treats. For people who are not healthy and whose daily diet is based on highly processed, nutrient-poor "junk", there may be little resilience to draw upon. In fact, people who have lived on such a diet frequently walk a tightrope, with their health fluctuating between good days and bad days based on an ever-changing list of factors.

What has happened, however, is that we have become "immoderate" in our thinking, expectations and our actions. We have made celebrations out of Friday night, Wednesday night, Saturday night and any other day or night that we can even remotely justify. We have created a need to celebrate the good report card, the birthday, the Little League win and even just getting through the week. We have created a culture of almost non-stop feast days and a subconscious need for repeated rewards. So while we speak of moderation, we frequently practice just the opposite. For many, the recitation of "all things in moderation" can be accurately translated to: "I want this food now, and I am going to eat it no matter what anyone says". The term "moderation" has become a deceptive cover to mask indulgence. Being honest with ourselves is a critical step to regaining our health, power and personal integrity and doing justice to our lives.

3. A calorie is a calorie

This myth is a big one. In fact, it is huge. It arose from the early days of dietitian training and is closely tied to calories-in-minus-calories-burned-equals-your-weight school of thought. Sadly, to the detriment of many, this myth is actively promoted today in dietetics. For a calorimeter in a laboratory setting, this concept is accurate, but such is not the case in biology. In the human body, how the body handles the calorie and what that calorie brings with it is more important than the quantity of calories. This belief has created a generation of people obsessed with caloric value even at the expense of nutrition. The evidence that calories are not the total answer to weight control can also be found in people you already know. It is the teenage boy or girl who can eat voluminous amounts of food, yet not gain an ounce. It is your uncle Ted who eats what he wants without showing any abdominal "spare-tire". And how do we explain this phenomenon to ourselves and to others? We say, "Well, it's their metabolism". The caloric approach to weight has been a colossal failure, and the frustrated souls who wander from one starvation diet to another are testament to the bankruptcy of the idea.

This concept is rooted deeply in people's minds and may take the form of the idea that you can eat a serving of greasy French fries as long as you "compensate" by working out at the gym for an extra half hour to "burn off" those calories. This belief supposes that there is a barter system governed by calories, and that if you simply make the trade, then all will be well. No, 50 calories from pretzels are not the same as 50 calories from spinach. You cannot exchange 100 calories of ice cream for 100 calories of broccoli and call it even.

Here is another example. Consider the notion that having a breakfast splurge at the local pancake house on Sunday morning. You decide to order a ten-ounce glass of orange juice accompanied by a platter-sized plate of pancakes doing the backstroke in high-fructose imitation maple syrup dusted with powdered sugar and declare it okay because it's only once a week and you plan on going to the gym later that day anyway. This scenario is a combination of the moderation myth and the calorie-is-a-calorie myth.

And what about that Sunday pancake bonanza? Well, assuming that every meal you eat after that is totally healthy and nutritious, it will take four to five days for your body to recover from that Sunday splurge. That means your body takes until Thursday to recover from the stress of the huge carbohydrate infusion. And by Thursday, well, it's only a couple of days until Sunday again!

Understanding that food can be analyzed on several levels is also important. At the most basic, macro level, we can measure the amount of fats, carbohydrates and proteins, which serve as the building blocks for repair and energy functions. At the next level, we can measure the quantity of specific vitamins, minerals and essential fatty acids that a specific food contains. These elements are necessary to support the enzymatic processes that make metabolism possible. But there is also a third level, which is the "informational" content that a food provides. Yes, food also provides information to cells and speaks to the genes. Of the thousands and thousands of plant compounds called phytonutrients, we now understand that these compounds influence our physiology in profound ways, even if the substances are only present in minute amounts. So, revisiting our comparison of 100 calories worth of ice cream versus broccoli, the two are vastly different nutritionally and informationally. The caloric value is almost a relative distraction.

4. A healthy diet can still include all the foods you like

This is another interesting concept that probably originates from the "everything in moderation" belief. Over the years, I saw people with persistent, chronic illness who emphatically voiced their desires and intentions to get well naturally but then proceeded to tell me what they really liked and had to include in their new, supposedly healthy diet. Clearly, what they had been eating and doing therapeutically had not translated into improved health thus far, but they also indicated they did not want to change very much either. It was as if they believed I could help them rearrange the foods they liked on their plate so the foods would now, suddenly, become healthy.

When you are working to improve your health, positively influencing your physiology multiples times per day is extremely advantageous. Biology changes with repeated signals to do so. Thus people working to recover their health typically respond better when they adhere to eating the high nutrient density foods that provide what they need at on a frequent basis. This approach is typically regarded as the "therapeutic diet" and is designed with the intent to move the physiological set point to a different level. The therapeutic diet is necessarily different from a "maintenance diet", which may be more relaxed and flexible once healing and resilience are achieved. The greatest challenges are observed when people's individual eating habits have been so distorted and unhealthy for so many years that even a maintenance diet feels like an impossibly strict regime. Without a recalibration of their understanding, these people will tend to struggle with feelings of deprivation and limitation.

5. My cravings indicate what my body truly needs

Our bodies do have incredible innate intelligence that is always directed to self-regulation and self-repair. Those with developed intuition can be guided to resources and solutions that were not the result of linear, left-brain analysis. However, I have rarely seen cravings as an indicator of that higher intelligence. The concept is an attractive one, but it is rarely true. Two examples come to mind.

The first example is chocolate. Over the years, I had many clients who would confidently declare that their affinity for chocolate was an indication that they needed something in that chocolate to be healthy. Frequently, they had looked up the nutritional analysis for chocolate and concluded, "Well, it must be the magnesium I really need and my body is craving the magnesium". Interested in exploring that further, I would ask, so what kind of chocolate do you crave? Of course, each client had their "favorite". To that I would reply, if it were something in chocolate your body was craving, then you should like plain, unsweetened, 100% chocolate, for that is just chocolate. Well, it did not take long for a quick look of discomfort to flash across their face as they realized that it was not the magnesium that was the draw, but the magic of the sweet-fat flavor sensation that made chocolate a craved food. If I said, "Okay, eat some plain, unsweetened organic chocolate every night", then the craving quickly lost its power. This example illustrates how we can misinterpret biological signals and draw incorrect conclusions.

The second example involves peanut butter. In the early years of clinical nutrition, clients would often cite peanut butter as a favorite protein food (although it was frequently complemented with highly processed sugary jam on white bread). Many claimed they loved peanut butter, often with the same interpretation that their bodies craved something in the peanut butter, such as the protein or amino acids, so naturally they gave in and ate it. Invariably, the peanut butter product they ate was really a peanut butter spread (you know the big names here), comprised of roughly 1/3 sugar, 1/3 cheap hydrogenated oil and 1/3 peanut butter. When I suggest switching to pure, 100% organic peanut butter with no added sugar or cheap oils, the magical desire for peanut butter quickly disappeared.

Food processors spend millions and millions of dollars devising ways to tease and trick your taste buds. Fats carry flavor, and if you mix fats (oils) and sugar, then you have a very powerful taste combination, such as "regular" peanut butter or chocolate products. Many food additives are intentionally designed to not only enhance taste but also to be addictive so you will purchase the product repeatedly in order to achieve the repeated mood modification effects. (See the book *Excitotoxins: The Taste that Kills* by Dr. Russell Blaylock for more information on this topic.)

Cravings may also be an expression of the desire for any food or substance that modifies our mood. When feeling distressed, stressed, depressed, anxious, melancholy or any other unpleasant emotional state, we instinctively search for ways to ameliorate that discomfort. Some people go shopping, some use alcohol, marijuana or other drugs, some turn to sex and other use the easy choice: food and drink. Anything that modifies our mood has the potential to create dependence. There is also a peculiar somewhat paradoxical phenomenon referred to as "allergy-addiction" where we crave the very food to which we have become sensitive or allergic, again, usually due to its mood modifying effects. This concept was pioneered may years ago by forward-thinking pediatricians like Dr. Doris Rapp, who said that if you wanted to know what your child was most likely allergic (or sensitive) to, look at their five top favorite foods. This idea was an invaluable insight that I found to be very helpful in working with many children and adults.

Our honorable but somewhat simplistic notion that our common cravings are an expression of our higher intelligence is little match for the sensory misdirection created by modern food chemists working in the lab. Do we have a higher intelligence that can direct us to a healthy variety of nutritious foods? I say, emphatically, *yes*. When we are healthy, in balance and dealing with naturally grown, unprocessed foods, I believe we can listen to that voice with confidence.

6. Breakfast foods

If we were to examine the origins of the current concept of a breakfast in the US, we would see a stark difference between the US and many other, non-Westernized nations. There is also a difference between pre-WWII and post-WWII America. The power of advertising changed the concept of breakfast in the minds of Americans in only a few years. For example, the notion of orange juice as a breakfast food was the result of a conscious marketing campaign by Florida orange growers. Juice was originally served in a small, 2-oz. "juice glass". Later, as the concept was repeated and exploited, the size of that juice glass grew. Boxed cereals also appeared post-WWII. Later came grab-and-go carb foods, such as croissants and muffins. The concept of bacon and eggs as a hearty breakfast was the advertising brainchild of Edward Bernays. In an effort to help increase the sale of bacon, he conducted a survey of physicians asking what kind of breakfast they recommended. The physicians responded by saying they recommended eating a "hearty breakfast". Bernays took their response and sent it out to 5,000 physicians, along with publicity touting "bacon and eggs" as a hearty breakfast. Voila! Bacon and eggs!

So, what makes any one food a breakfast food, lunch food or dinner food? The answer is not a biological one, but one of habit, culture and conditioning. When you break free of this limiting belief, meals have more flexibility and interest. In doing so, you have the freedom to eat that which is healthy and satisfying regardless of the time of day or the name of the meal.

7. If it weren't proven safe and effective, then my doctor wouldn't prescribe it

This statement is a nice idea, and it would be even nicer if actually true. A cursory review of medical history tends to reveal another story, often forgotten and seldom discussed. The point here is not to condemn modern medicine. All fields move forward with incomplete information, usually based on ideas and theories that may be proven wrong at a later date. All professionals in all fields struggle with this issue. Such is life without a crystal ball. The point is made to underscore the importance of doing your own assessment, both logical and intuitive, rather than making a decision to simply trust what is being offered. X-rays for acne, prefrontal lobotomies for depression, electroconvulsive shock for depression, bleedings for fever, Calomel for infections, arsenic for syphilis, eggs are good, eggs are bad—not an inspiring track record.

The Office of Technology Assessment (OTA), a branch of the United States Congress, with the help of an advisory board of eminent university faculty, published a report in the late 1970s that reviewed questions about what had been proven "safe" or "effective" in current medical methods. Based on their research, they concluded that "… only 10 to 20 percent of all procedures currently used in medical practice have been shown to be efficacious by controlled trial." That means that 80% to 90% of medical procedures routinely performed are unproven. (I have placed the reference for this in Appendix B)

The OTA repeated their review of medical procedures roughly twenty years later, when they compared medical technology in eight countries (Australia, Canada, France, Germany, the Netherlands, Sweden, the UK and the US). In 1995, they issued their report (see Appendix B for information), which again stated that few medical procedures in the US had been subject to clinical trials. They also reported that US infant mortality was high and overall life expectancy low compared to the other developed countries. Shortly after this report was released, the office was disbanded and no further studies were performed.

Furthermore, in the United States, the Food and Drug Administration (FDA) has the sole responsibility to approve new drugs for human use, ostensibly based on their safety and efficacy. So why then is the third-leading cause of death in the United States death from prescription drugs that are properly prescribed by licensed physicians with full oversight in a hospital setting? According to conservative estimates that are published in mainstream medical journals and listed on the FDA's own web site, on average 106,000 people die from prescription medications *each year*. That figure represents 1.06 million Americans every ten years. There is no outrage. There is no uproar. You probably were never told. So what should patients believe about the relative safety of FDA-approved drugs? What should patients believe about the safety of drugs prescribed by physicians for purposes not approved by the FDA, the so-called off-label uses? There is good reason why patients and their families need to do their own homework on any drug that is being prescribed before risking becoming another statistic.

Having some understanding of these important facts helps us reason through difficult medical decisions and avoid the rigid, sometimes fanatical devotion to treatments that may not stand the test of time. The larger concept at hand reminds me of Andrew Carnegie's statement: "He that cannot reason is a fool. He that will not is a bigot. He that dare not is a slave."

Part V

The Conceptual Myths in Health and Disease

Chapter 23

Conceptual Myth #1: Normal or Common

"An error does not become truth by reason of multiplied propagation, nor does the truth become error because nobody will see it." – Mahatma Gandhi

One of the most interesting concepts in health and medicine is the idea of "normal". What is normal? Who decides what normal is? Why does the definition of normal keep changing? Would being considered normal when it comes to your health a step forward or a step backward? People living in Westernized societies with a reliance on highly processed foods and pharmaceutical interventions to block symptoms have been induced to accept the premise that with aging, one should view certain illnesses as normal. While it is true that arthritis, asthma, diabetes, dementia do occur more frequently with advancing age in some populations, it is not true in all populations.

As participants in society, we witness the health of the other people in our personal worlds: relatives, family, friends, co-workers, people we meet socially or the waitress in a coffee house. We encounter people with all manner of health issues, such as obesity, joint pain, migraine, asthma and so forth, and we make assumptions and conclusions about the frequency of these conditions. Interacting with your medical practitioner may further add to our familiarity with illness. Through all of these interactions, we begin to see that certain conditions appear frequently and because they do, we are inclined to conclude that they are "normal". Here is a simpler example. Let's suppose that you live in a northern latitude location such as Minnesota in the US, or Denmark, and it is January. There is an epidemic of flu, and it seems that everyone now has the flu. Is it normal or common to have the flu? It is common. As people become increasingly immunocompromised, illnesses such as flu spread further into populations, and the number of people who become ill increases. But does that mean you should expect to be ill? Even in the most deadly plagues in history, not everyone succumbed. Some portion of the population remained healthy and survived. Are the survivors the aberration? Is having good immunity to be expected, or is illness to be expected? It can be argued that in a healthy population of well-nourished people who have learned to take care of themselves and practice preventive medicine, such mass epidemics would be rare or limited in their scope. But prevention is neither taught nor encouraged in Western cultures, and there is certainly no profit in remaining well.

If the rate of heart disease, arthritis, autoimmune disease and cancer increases in a society (as they are doing), *should* we redefine normal to be the same as increased incidence of the disease? Should we then also change our expectations about our chances of having the disease? Even if the odds now suggest that there is a 1 in 3 chance you will have cancer in your lifetime, does that mean you *will* have cancer and that having cancer is normal? Thirty years ago, the incidence of autism was roughly 1 in 25,000 children. It is now (according to the CDC as reported in 2012) roughly 1 in 88 children. Some researchers predict that in the next ten years, the incidence may change to 1 in 10. When it reaches 1 in 10 or 1 in 5, will we then redefine having a non-communicative child as the new normal? Whether you look at infant mortality, longevity, cancer rates, diabetes, or other markers, what you will see after a careful examination of the evidence is that when normal is periodically redefined, it does not mean healthier. When it comes to my health, I do not want it to be normal! It appears that Albert Einstein wasn't especially fond of being considered normal either and is quoted as having said: "No one is remembered for being normal".

It would be easy to assert and support an argument that the prevalence of these chronic conditions represents a failure of not only modern medicine, but also in addressing issues at the causative level. Perhaps that perspective will shock us into looking for causes rather than treating symptoms.

Chapter 24

Conceptual Myth #2: Genes Control Your Health

Its been nearly 60 years since the modern discovery of DNA and our understanding of exactly how it affects our health continues to change. And while many people will talk about DNA, few understand how it works.

Author and commentator James Le Fanu, MD, in his piece entitled "Science's Dead End", speaks of a disconcerting surprise that arose upon the completion of the human genome project. Biologists were shocked to discover that there was a "near equivalence" of some 20,000 genes across the spectrum of life forms, ranging from simple worms to complex humans. Dr. Le Fanu goes on to say that it was "no less disconcerting to learn that the human genome is virtually interchangeable with that of both the mouse and our primate cousins..." and that the genome could not explain "why the fly has six legs, a pair of wings and a dot-sized brain and that we should have two arms, two legs and a mind capable of comprehending the history of our universe..."

But I think Dr. Fanu's most telling observation is one that really shifts our perspective:

> At a time when cosmologists can reliably infer what happened in the first few minutes of the birth of the universe, and geologists can measure the movements of

continents to the nearest centimetre, it seems extraordinary that geneticists can't tell us why humans are so different from flies, and neuroscientists are unable to clarify how we recall a telephone number.

With the discovery of DNA by Watson and Crick in 1954, scientists and medical researchers had a new understanding and a model to explain the appearance of various traits, diseases and conditions in related family members. Austrian scientist and Augustinian friar Gregor Mendel discovered the science of genetics long ago. It is distinction that was only awarded to him posthumously since, as with many scientific advances, he research ran afoul of the thinking of his day. In the second half of the twentieth century, the gene concept of disease quickly gained wide acceptance, probably in part due to the effect of lifting any sense of responsibility from the patient in the initiation or evolution of their condition and also, no doubt, due to the specter of huge profits from future gene therapy. Since a genetic condition implied that there was no control or alternative to the inevitable disease, the victim mentality in disease was greatly strengthened.

Recent discoveries, however, strongly suggest that genes play a far less controlling role than once assumed. Genes do not turn themselves on or off spontaneously, There is a protein sleeve that covers the genetic sequence, allowing or disallowing it to be "read". In early DNA research, this protein was referred to as "junk protein" and discarded because scientists did not know what it was for. Now, it appears the protein is the controlling mechanism whereby genes become activated or silenced. But what controls the protein sleeve? These controlling factors are called "epigenetic", meaning "above" the genes. As it turns out, there are many epigenetic factors that affect gene expression, such as Vitamin D, toxins, emotions, stress and methylation status, to name just a few. In fact, some researchers believe that Vitamin D3 may influence the expression of up to 3,000 genes, which may not sound significant until you realize that as humans, we only have roughly 25,000 genes.

This brings up an incredible example how wrong a scientific "fact" can be. When I was a student in undergraduate and graduate school, the reigning dogma in biology and genetics class was "one gene, one protein", meaning that one single gene was responsible for the production of one single protein, a very simple concept on its face. Students simply had to know this phrase and recite it upon command. The belief that genes controlled our health was so strong that the concept was referred to as "The Central Dogma" right in the biology books! When we examine the meaning of the pivotal word "dogma", we find the definition (according to dictionary.com) to be: "prescribed doctrine proclaimed as unquestionably true by a particular group" and "a settled or established opinion, belief, or principle". Sounds a bit like a religion, doesn't it?

Because scientists believed in the one gene, one protein concept and knew that a human has roughly 100,000 unique proteins and approximately 20,000 regulatory genes, then they concluded that there should be at least 120,000 genes within the 23 pairs of chromosomes. But nature is not without a sense of humor. To the shock of researchers at the conclusion of the human genome project (concluded in 2003), approximately 25,000 genes were discovered, not the 120,000 or more genes they expected! How could the estimate of the best scientists of the day be off by almost 80%? Such an error is not a near miss! This discovery created quite a controversy, at least quietly. The problem was that the complexity of the human, with 50 trillion cells, could not be explained by the genetic findings and the one gene, one protein dogma. The fruit fly contains 15,000 genes. The microscopic roundworm known as *Caenorhabditis elegans* has a genome consisting of nearly 24,000 genes, but has a body consisting of only 969 cells and a rudimentary brain comprised of a scant 302 cells! As it turns out, each gene can create hundreds or even thousands of different variations of a protein, based upon how that gene is expressed. The factors that influence the expression of a gene are the epigenetic factors we speak of now.

Knowing that genes can be turned on also allows for the concept that genes can be silenced, or turned off. To have a gene that predisposes you for developing breast cancer, colon cancer or pancreatic cancer is one thing. With the current belief that only five to ten percent of all cancers are genetic in origin, how do we explain the roughly 1 in 3 appearance of cancer in Western societies? Even for those cancers that do have a genetic basis, this is not a cause for despair. To have that gene silenced by epigenetic factors means that genetically predisposed cancer will not occur.

It is indeed curious that people hold such a strong inclination—even desire—to believe in the theory of genetic control: that genes control our health. Perhaps our belief in genetics is genetic? But that inclination does not change the reality that genes are not the rigid controllers of future health. If they were, none of use would be living *our* lives. We would all be living the lives and legacy of our ancestors with no hope for change or relief. Fortunately, such is not the case, but believing it puts you into a prison and limits your true potential and power to heal.

This new biology is the essence of a new, empowering paradigm within the science. It will be interesting to see how the vanguard for the "old biology" resists this emerging paradigm. There are some excellent resources listed in the Resources Appendix that can provide the reader with additional information. As science zigs and zags toward greater understanding, it does bump into, what appear to be, contradictions in the facts. Writer Ayn Rand summarized this experience when she admonished: "Contradictions do not exist. Whenever you think you are facing a contradiction, check your premises. You will find that one of them is wrong."

Chapter 25

Conceptual Myth #3: The Illusion of Side Effects

Modern medicine is based largely on pharmacological and surgical interventions. Since the late 1800s, drugs have been increasingly relied upon for everything from pain relief to sexual pleasure. While drugs do have their place, to be sure, they often become the "quick fix" to suppress symptoms in busy people who are out of touch with their bodies and emotions.

Drugs are not without the potential for creating undesirable effects. If you wanted to understand what effects one might experience when a particular chemical substance is ingested, you could look that chemical up in a toxicology book. Wikipedia defines toxicology as follows: "a branch of biology, chemistry, and medicine concerned with the study of the adverse effects of chemicals on living organisms. It is the study of symptoms, mechanisms, treatments and detection of poisoning, especially the poisoning of people."

Let's say you are going to do some indoor painting, and you read on the label of the paint can that it contains xylene. You are concerned about xylene and its effects, so you decide do some online research to understand more about the toxicology of xylene. Xylene is commonly used as a solvent and, as a crude oil derivative, it is foreign to your body. In this example, you are likely to inhale the xylene, rather than ingest it. So, if you were to obtain this information from the US

Occupational Safety and Health Administration (OSHA) it would, in part, show the following:

OSHA: * Signs and symptoms of exposure

1. Acute exposure: The signs and symptoms of acute exposure to xylene include headache, fatigue, irritability, lassitude, nausea, anorexia, flatulence, irritation of the eyes, nose, and throat, and motor incoordination and impairment of equilibrium. Flushing, redness of the face, a sensation of increased body heat, increased salivation, tremors, dizziness, confusion, and cardiac irritability have also been reported.

2. Chronic exposure: The signs and symptoms of chronic exposure to xylene may include conjunctivitis; dryness of the nose, throat, and skin; dermatitis; and kidney and liver damage.

In all likelihood, if you were exposed, you would not experience every symptom that exposure to xylene *could* produce. Your nutritional status, liver detoxification pathway functionality, underlying genetic variations, prior total toxic body burden and many other factors would all temper the manifestation of which symptoms are emphasized and which are minimized. All of the symptoms listed are the *direct effects* of a toxic exposure to xylene, not *side effects*.

The majority of prescription and over-the-counter drugs used today are foreign synthetic chemicals. The exceptions are the bio-identical hormones and other so-called biologicals that are sometimes prescribed. So, whether you are talking about acetaminophen, or simvastatin, or escitalopram oxalate, you are speaking of synthetic compounds that are ingested by people to create or produce some effect. If you were to look up any of these compounds, you would see, as with any toxicology reference, a list of effects that this compound can produce, depending on the individual and the dose taken.

When you look over the list, you will notice that there are one or two specific effects that we *like and desire* and a number of effects that we *do not like*. Because you ingested this chemical compound for the effect you like and desire, we call that the "therapeutic effect", which is the reason why the chemical compound, now called a drug, was prescribed. But you will also experience some of the effects that you do not like, again depending on the dose and your particular sensitivity. Those are also the effects of the compound, but because they are not the ones we desire, they are called "side effects". The difference is really both a phenomenon of the intention behind why the chemical compound was prescribed (intent) and of marketing by Big Pharma. Such a change in perspective can totally alter how we look at drugs and their impact on our physiology. All of the effects, both the desired ones and the undesired ones, are the *effects* of the drug. So if we now return to the example of xylene above, we notice that one of the *effects* is increased salivation. If for some strange reason, xylene were prescribed to a person with dry mouth syndrome, the "increased salivation" might be considered a "therapeutic benefit", could it not? Or, perhaps to a person who chronically feels cold, the effect of "a sensation of increased body heat" might be seen as a therapeutic benefit, would it not? But would the other effects experienced be properly called "side effects" or merely "the effects"?

Whether you ingested acetaminophen for the pain in your ankle or the headache you developed from not eating on time, the fact is that each and every cell in your body was dosed with that acetaminophen and had to deal with it. Unlike the smart biological compounds that are produced and used within our bodies, these chemicals are dumb, because they are unable to target only the symptom that brought you to the physician's office. Neither the drug nor your body knows *why* you took it or *where* it was intended to go. Of course it creates symptoms you don't want!

Altering our perception of how drugs work can help us make better decisions in healthcare. The goal is good medicine—medicine that is safe and effective for the issues we seek to address. This discussion is not to say that all drugs are "bad" or that they are never appropriate. Drugs *can* be live saving. If you had major surgery to replace a hip, you may certainly want to avail yourself of modern pain medication while you repair and recover. If you are in crisis, conventional medication may absolutely be your best choice, at least for the moment. The question becomes more complex when facing chronic conditions and illnesses that result from unhealthy lifestyle patterns, poor food choices, uncontrolled stress, environmental exposures and the like. We usually get ourselves into difficulties with our desire for a quick fix and our impatience to make symptoms magically and suddenly disappear.

Chapter 26

Conceptual Myth #4: Modern Medicine or Good Medicine

For decades, Americans have enjoyed a high standard of living and long life expectancy. There has also been a strong though rapidly weakening belief that medical care in the US is not only the most sophisticated medical care in the world, but also that it is "the best". This belief has been deeply ingrained in the American psyche and reinforced at all levels of society. If by "best" you mean "most expensive", then you are 100% correct. If you define "best" by the health of the American people, then another conclusion would be reached.

It is necessary to ask why people in general, and Americans in particular, invest so much trust in modern medicine. What results, outcomes or national statistics does one point to support such a belief? The question is actually a very important one, for it affects how we view the development of diseases. If you believe that you can simply live life the way you want, eat and drink what you like, ignore your own biological requirements and then when things break modern medicine will fix you, then there is little incentive for prevention.

Author and commentator James Le Fanu, MD offers this perspective in *The Rise and Fall of Modern Medicine:*

Medicine has become the most visible symbol of the fulfillment of the great Enlightenment Project where scientific progress would vanquish the twin perils of ignorance and disease to the benefit of all. And yet the more powerful and prestigious it has become, the greater the impetus to extend its influence further, resulting in the progressive 'medicalisation' of people's lives to no good purpose... this takes many forms from the over investigation and over treatment of minor symptoms to the inappropriate use of life-sustaining technologies, anxiety mongering about trivial (or non existent) threats to health and people's everyday lives, and the propagation of unreasonable expectations about what the current state of medical research can reasonably be expected to achieve.

There are drugs to lower your cholesterol and drugs to increase your libido, drugs for anxiety and drugs for depression, drugs for diarrhea and drugs for constipation, drugs for hyperthyroid and more drugs for hypothyroid. You understand the concept. It is very much what I refer to as a "bumper and fender" approach to care. Despite all the advances in science and physics, modern medicine remains locked in a Newtonian, clockwork, mechanical model wherein the "everything is separate" perspective is dominant. In most cases, medicine does not work *with* the body at all. Rather, it works *on* the body as if each of the individual organs and systems were separate from the rest of the body. You see a cardiologist for the heart. A rheumatologist for your joints. An ENT for your ears, nose and throat. A dentist for your mouth. A podiatrist for your feet. Yes, they better stay within their own defined professional turf lest they step into another specialist's domain. Heavens, they would be practicing integrated medicine!

If you have not looked at the statistics of what modern medicine has done and is doing to the population, then there are a couple of well researched and documented reviews that will greatly shorten your research time. One is entitled "Death by Medicine" by Gary Null, PhD, et al.. This report will provide you with the statistics, references and commentary to guide you to better understand this complex issue. The other article, a very conservative review published in the *Journal of the American Medical Association* by Barbara Starfield, MD, MPH will also add to your understanding. (The full citation for the Starfield article is located in the Resources Appendix) If you read either of these articles and take the statistics I quote below seriously, you will need no additional incentive to begin actively taking responsibility for your own health. As I have said previously, this book is not about bashing the medical system or the hard-working physicians and nurses who do the best they can from within the paradigm they were taught. It is about gaining an understanding about a system that purports to be based on scientific data and objective research. So what do the statistics have to say?

- The number of people who die each year due to physician-prescribed pharmaceuticals administered within the control and monitoring of a hospital setting is conservatively estimated at 106,000 per year. That calculates to 1.06 million deaths per ten years;

- The number of people having in-hospital, adverse reactions to prescription drugs is 2.2 million per year;

- The number of unnecessary antibiotic prescriptions written for viral infections is roughly twenty million per year;

- The number of unnecessary medical and surgical procedures performed is 7.5 million per year;

- The number of people unnecessarily hospitalized annually is 8.9 million;

- The number of deaths due to medical errors is 980,000 over ten years;

- The costs of adverse drug reactions to society are more than $136 billion annually, greater than the total cost of cardiovascular or diabetic care;

- The ten-year death rate due to malnutrition is 1.09 million patients;

- The number of deaths due to nosocomial (hospital-acquired) infections is 880,000 over ten years; and

- Based on the available data, the authors of "Death by Medicine" estimated that the total number of iatrogenic (physician caused) deaths for a ten-year period is 7.8 million, which is greater than the total of all casualties from all the wars fought by the US throughout its entire history.

Unfortunately, the list goes on.

What about life expectancy? Isn't the US still near the top?

In 2010, the latest US life expectancy statistics were published in *Health Affairs* and showed that life expectancy had dropped, making the US now 50th in the world. A full 49 countries have longer life expectancies than the US. This figure is down from 24th in 1999. In 1950, the US was 5th among leading industrialized nations with respect to female life expectancy at birth. Only Sweden, Norway, Australia and the Netherlands ranked higher. The last available measure of female life expectancy ranked the US as 46th in the world.

What about infant mortality rates? The 2011 data from the UN has the US at 34th in the world, with Singapore, Iceland and Japan being #1, #2 and #3 on the list. The infant mortality rate is defined as the number of deaths of infants under one year old per 1,000 live births. The US Centers for Disease Control says that the infant mortality rate is a key indicator of overall health standards and health care. The US ranked behind Macau, Cyprus, Croatia and Cuba.

Where does the US rank highest? The US ranks number one in the world on dollars spent on medical care.

So, here is the question that needs to be asked: if Americans are the beneficiaries of all this advanced medical research, medications, vaccines, medical screenings, high-technology CT scans and MRIs, then shouldn't there be some evidence *somewhere* of improving health? Shouldn't Americans expect that at least some of the billions and billions of dollars spent on medical research translate into some measurable improvement in life?

It does not, and I would suggest that it could not. The fact is, the healthcare industry is in all actuality a disease-care industry that has focused on two areas: testing/screenings and treatments. When you look at US healthcare more carefully, treatment for many conditions today is directed toward managing the condition: managing your diabetes, managing your MS symptoms, managing your fibromyalgia, managing your rheumatoid arthritis. Managing, not reversing. Managing means dependence. There is little talk of effective cures or even an expectation that you will get substantially better. There is even less talk about prevention. Even your high blood pressure is called "essential hypertension"! Essential? Why is it that we have a "walk for the cure" (which really means treatment) rather than a "walk for the cause"?

Physicians will tell you that the foundation of modern medicine is science and objective evidence generated by research studies. The research, they will tell you, is what distinguishes supposedly real medicine from all of that anecdotal, natural medicine stuff. So, what about all that research published in all of those allegedly prestigious medical journals? Within the higher ranks of modern medicine, the fact that so many of these studies are either faked, contrived or conducted by think-tanks funded entirely by the pharmaceutical industry to support preconceived conclusions is no secret. Physicians are enticed to be listed as a researcher or author on a study that they did not perform and did not author. In fact, the problem is so severe that Marcia Angell, MD, who served as editor of *The New England Journal of Medicine* for two decades, resigned in protest over the issue. In her statement, she said:

> It is simply no longer possible to believe much of the clinical research that is published, or to rely on the judgment of trusted physicians or authoritative medical guidelines.

Dr. Angell also commented on how drugs are tested on humans in clinical trials. She states:

> Before a new drug can enter the market, its manufacturer must sponsor clinical trials to show the Food and Drug Administration that the drug is safe and effective, usually as compared with a placebo or dummy pill. The results of all the trials (there may be many) are submitted to the FDA, and if one or two trials are positive—that is, they show effectiveness without serious risk—the drug is usually approved, even if all the other trials are negative.

In a May 2009 article appearing in *The New York Review of Books*, author Helen Epstein had this observation in speaking about the corruption of medical science:

> ..... peer-reviewed articles in medical journals can be crucial in influencing multimillion- and sometimes multibillion-dollar spending decisions. It would be surprising if conflicts of interest did not sometimes compromise editorial neutrality, and in the case of medical research, the sources of

bias are obvious. Most medical journals receive half or more of their income from pharmaceutical company advertising and reprint orders....

While the endemic corruption of medical science is a huge concern, it is not the entire problem. Individually and collectively as a society, we transferred our faith and trust, and hence our power, to this system in the hopes that it would provide the answers and rescue us. In transferring that power, we abdicated our responsibility to ourselves to foster and maintain our own health. We looked to others and surrendered our power to them in the vain hope that a pill or procedure would safely, effortlessly and quickly reverse what we have done to ourselves. Prevention, as espoused by the medical system, has been distilled down to a quaint though useless slogan: "Eat right, exercise and see your doctor". Does anyone really think that is useful?

Ultimately, the answer is clear. In order to get different results, we must change what we do and how we think. As Albert Einstein once said: "Insanity is doing the same thing over and over but expecting different results". *You* are responsible for your health. You have the power through conscious choice or by ignorance and neglect to create the level of health that you desire. You may choose to enlist the assistance of one or more professionals who are willing to share the benefit of their training and experience. But ultimately we must reclaim the power, authority and responsibility for our path.

Chapter 27

Conceptual Myth #5: The Balanced Diet is All You Need

This very appealing argument exists in several variations, and it is usually asserted by professionals who work within the conventional medical-pharmaceutical paradigm. The origins of this belief can be traced back to the early days of nutritional research and simple dietetics. In those days, research involved the identification of overt nutritional deficiency states, such as scurvy, beriberi, rickets or pellagra, which are conditions that can be tied to an overt deficiency of a single nutrient. When the deficient nutrient was added back into the diet of the deficient person, their symptoms reversed. Thus, it was easy to conclude that a binary, deficient/not-deficient state existed, as expressed by the symptoms. In fact, an entire line of thinking was established on this concept, which gave birth to the Recommended Daily Allowance (RDA) in the US and similar guidelines in other countries. This project was initially sponsored by the US Government and later assumed by the US Food and Nutrition Board, which is a committee of the National Academy of Sciences' National Research Council. The Board is a composite of researchers, academicians and others, although most have strong ties to the processed food industry.

As the Board defines them, the RDAs are "the levels of intake of essential nutrients considered, in the judgment of the Food and

Nutrition Board on the basis of available scientific knowledge, to be adequate to meet the known nutritional needs of practically all healthy persons."

Can you see a few problems in that definition? Let me repeat the definition with the problem words underlined:

"...the levels of intake of <u>essential</u> nutrients considered, in the <u>judgment</u> of the Food and Nutrition Board on the basis of <u>available scientific</u> knowledge, to be <u>adequate</u> to meet the <u>known</u> nutritional needs of <u>practically</u> all <u>healthy</u> persons."

Talk about wiggle room in a statement! What about the benefit of nutrients they do not consider essential at this moment in time? Also, the judgment of a committee usually means a vote; was the vote unanimous, or did the members disagree among themselves? What if their judgment is biased toward their supporting companies or research funding? What about the scientific information that was not available? Why wasn't it available? Who did the search for available information and decided it was complete? Why the reliance on scientific knowledge? There is a lot that science cannot prove or has not even tried to prove. What about common sense? Is that included? How much "science" has to be done, and by whom, before the information they derive is regarded as knowledge? Even more telling is that the definition speaks of *adequate* levels of nutrients, not *optimal*. Adequate for whom? Teens? Pregnant women? Post-surgical patients? The elderly? People under stress? And what are known nutritional needs? What about those nutritional needs that have not been studied yet? Who is conducting the studies? Who is funding the studies? Is a nutrient unimportant because it has attracted no research funding yet? When will new information be regarded as valuable, and who gets to decide this? The government? Food industry researchers? And lastly, the RDAs are meant to cover practically all, not all, but most, healthy people. Who are these healthy people? Can you find any?

Define "healthy". In Western cultures, if you are taking an antacid for your heartburn, a statin for your cholesterol, a stool-softener for your bowels, and an SSRI for your depression, but are not outwardly bleeding, oozing, seeping, sneezing or expectorating and can walk and talk well enough to go to work, you generally regarded as healthy, are you not? How many drugs can you be on and still be included in the category of "healthy"? Do you think three percent of the population is not taking drugs? On further scrutiny, it would appear that the RDAs really do not apply to many real people, just some statistical, theoretical model of a man or woman living an ideal life in a non-stressful world, eating only whole, unprocessed foods grown on nutrient-rich soils since birth and born from a mother who did the same!

As the fallacy of the RDAs became more widely appreciated, the concept of "optimal" nutrition has gained acceptance as being another quite different state. So, within the framework of biochemical individuality, a person could be in an overtly deficient state (with presenting symptoms of deficiency), in a state of "nutritional adequacy" (no classic symptoms of deficiency) or in a state of "optimal nutrition" wherein all nutrients were provided at levels ideally suited to optimize the physiological functioning of that specific and unique individual. This optimal state is unlikely to be achieved accidentally without an express purpose and plan to achieve it. Nevertheless, such a state is possible based on the development of sophisticated tests that can measure the genetic SNPs (single nucleotide polymorphisms) that account for individual variations in function and advanced functional tests that can evaluate multiple points in our physiology for evidence of interference and reduced functionality. This analysis would include tests for heavy metals, aberrations in mitochondrial energy function, defective methylation and detoxification function, toxic overload and more.

The balanced diet myth is hypothecated on the fictional notion that humans are somewhat homogeneous in their nutritional needs and that some sort of generally balanced diet can be devised that will work for most everyone. That hypothesis *might* be plausible if all we were considering only overt nutrient deficiency states.

The reality is, of course, quite to the contrary. For one, there is no agreement on what diet is best for each group of people: children, adolescents, adult pre-menopausal women, sedentary men, active men, highly stressed adults, people who drink alcohol and so on. We know that certain functions, such as specific liver enzyme systems involved in detoxifying various endogenous compounds, such as estrogens, can vary ten-fold from person to person. Further, if you look up carrots or raspberries in a food-nutrient table, typically the USDA table, it will tell you the nutritional content of carrots: the level of beta-carotene, Vitamin C, etc. But is it telling you about carrots grown in California, New York, Florida, Chile, Mexico or any of a number of different locations with different soil nutrient content? Plus, those analyses were completed and compiled *when*? 1946? We have an additional 60-plus years of farming since then, with only three nutrients added back to the soil to stimulate plant growth, not to replenish the soil. Yes, plants can generally grow well with only N (nitrogen), P (phosphorous) and K (potassium or potash). Humans need roughly 90 nutrients to enjoy robust health. The plants require just three. Can you tell which nutrients the plants have or are missing by looking at them? Unfortunately, you can't.

The problem has not gone unnoticed; it has simply been ignored. As far back as the 74th Congress of the United States, it was disclosed in hearing before Congress that 99% of Americans were deficient in organic trace minerals because of economics-based farming and agricultural practices that depleted soils and destroyed the complex, life-sustaining organic complexes within the soil. The result of this chronic mistreatment and mass over-farming of the soils has produced what was called "hollow crops", which are then used in producing "hollow foods", foods that look and taste good but fail to provide the organic nutrient complexes and trace minerals that are necessary for human health. Additionally, these farming practices provided for the ingestion of numerous toxic chemicals used by farmers to produce more yield from increasingly unhealthy soil. In Appendix A, I have reproduced the text of this Congressional report.

The fact of the matter is that our foods, even when grown organically, can vary enormously in their nutritive value. Aside from merely appeasing our hunger, some conventionally grown foods really are not worth eating from a nutrition perspective. Vegetables grown in one part of the world may test out with 1,100 parts per billion (ppb) of iodine compared to only 20 ppb when grown elsewhere. Conventionally processed cow's milk may contain from 360 ppb iodine down to zero and from 127 ppb iron down to nothing. Not all virgin land contains an ideal or optimal balance of nutrients to begin with, and our penchant for raping the soil in the name of continuous yields has not remedied the situation. Ironically, our current technology would allow us to test the soil each year and amend it based on what it is missing. We could optimize the nutrient content of the soil and of the plants that grow upon it. Whether people would pay more for these carrots or broccoli remains to be seen.

Believing in the myth of the balanced diet may spawn additional derivative myths that will alter your decisions, choices and behaviors. For example, if you eat a balanced diet, then supplementing with additional nutrients:

- is unnecessary;
- just creates expensive urine;
- is a waste of money;
- is unproven;
- creates toxicity; or
- is just taking more pills.

I do not know about you, but I really want so-called expensive urine—and expensive, high-quality kidneys, red blood cells and skin! Do you see the point? People who do not like taking medications or pills have sometimes been conditioned to think of nutritional supplements as also being pills. For some people, taking pills evokes an emotional image of being sick, and thus they have an instinctive aversion to doing so. Thus, the position of "Well, doctor, I only want to take four to five vitamin pills, not a bunch" may be taken, rather than the position of "Well, doctor, I will take what I need to take to correct the deficiencies that I previously had and then work toward optimal health."

Chapter 28

Conceptual Myth #6: Trust the Experts

Much of the complexity of modern society is a creation of man's mind. We have created complex systems, codes, rules, policies, legal requirements, deadlines and finances that few understand but all are compelled to deal with. Realistically, few people can or choose to become master of each of these areas in life, so we hire and delegate that expertise to others. Perhaps you have an accountant or investment advisor. You probably have a dentist and a physician. Others might rely upon a chiropractor or osteopath. In other cultures, you might have an herbalist or shaman. Whenever an area becomes exceedingly complex, we seem to develop supposed experts to help navigate the muddy waters.

For those blessed with truly good health, born from healthy genetic stock and instilled with healthy beliefs and attitudes during their early years, maintaining health is a comparatively easy task compared to the challenge of restoring one's health. An extensive body of information on nutrition, exercise and more is available that can guide healthy behaviors and habits.

The journey to improve your health, once compromised, varies greatly in the nature and complexity of what may be required. If you are not a physician, chiropractor or other person with extensive training in anatomy, physiology, biochemistry, endocrinology, pharmacology and the art of diagnosis, then you will likely require expert guidance from those with such training and knowledge. You may have to seek their advice and recommendations regarding diagnosis, treatment options, surgery, medications, potential outcomes and their experienced judgment as a professional. It would be foolhardy to not seek competent help and guidance when we do not have the knowledge and skills ourselves. And even if you did, nobody would recommend being doctor to yourself!

One of the key questions that will inevitably arise is how to relate to that external source of expertise. As I mentioned earlier in Part III, the traditional physician-patient relationship more closely mirrored the parent-child dynamic than that of a healthy adult-to-adult relationship. Patients were often quiet, obedient, did not ask many questions, infrequently asked for a second opinion and would hardly consider questioning the doctor's advice. For many reasons, that dynamic is changing, and people are choosing to do their own research and seek other points of view. Many physicians welcome the change and are happy to be relieved of such awesome god-like responsibilities.

In the parent-child dynamic, the patient frequently feels safe (or safer) because they have transferred the responsibility for the success or failure of the treatment to the physician. Understandably, if you do not know much about biology, anatomy or medications and do not wish to learn, then making decisions for yourself can be daunting. At some point in time, we will have to place our trust in someone that we feel can help us and guide us. Doing so does not mean we need to abdicate trust in ourselves and our own inner sense. The adult asks for help when needed but does not abdicate responsibility to the helper. I would think that physicians would welcome this change in dynamics with their patients, if for no other reason than to alleviate the over-allocated sense of responsibility that they have traditionally carried. Medical decisions and health decisions are usually not black and white, and science and our understanding are both constantly changing and always incomplete.

So how do you become an active partner—an adult—in the physician-patient dynamic? Fundamentally, you arrive at the realization that your life, health and future well-being is *your* responsibility. Yes, your physician, chiropractor, naturopath, clinical nutritionist or acupuncturist is there to help you and provide the benefit of their years of study, knowledge and experience, but the buck stops with you. It sounds scary, but it has always been that way anyway! Even when the patients prefers to shift responsibility to the physician, who pays the price when things go wrong? Who suffers from the adverse drug reaction, botched surgery, the nosocomial infection or the mercury in the vaccine? The patient, of course.

For those who cherish their health and consider themselves to be active participants in maintaining or improving their personal or family health, acquiring accurate, useful and largely unbiased information is a key. While the public library once filled this role, the Internet is now the information vehicle of choice. There, anyone can post an opinion, publish a book or host a video on almost any topic they wish. For many people, trying to sort through this sea of information and disinformation is analogous to trying to take a drink from a fire hose. This amount of information may at first appear to be a *big* negative, but, in reality, a free Internet with all of the challenges that come with it is far better for all than a censored one. Censorship, of course, is always promoted to allegedly protect you from those products, ideas and opinions that do not conform or support those interests who wish to exert the control. Recall the statement by John D. Rockefeller: "Competition is a sin." Hence, when you take a cross-section of what was is called "main stream media" and examine their so-called news stories, editorials and commercial sponsors, you can detect the bias quite easily. Yet there are still pockets of Americans, and presumably others around the world, who still cling to their belief (or maybe just want to believe) that these once-respected voices that commanded the attention of millions would never act against the best interests of their viewers. Of course. Take a look at just a few issues that mainstream voices oppose, either by direct attack, innuendo or by total silence:

- The use and benefit of organic foods;
- Community Supported Agriculture (CSA);
- The benefits of locally grown and vine-ripened foods;
- Nutritional supplementation;
- Fluoride-free drinking water;
- Natural medicine treatment methods;
- Generic and imported medicines;
- Home schooling;
- Respect for responsible choice in vaccination;
- Parental rights in raising their children; and
- Mandatory labeling of GMO foods.

This list just names a few. Why do these topics not receive positive attention in the media? You only have to follow the money trail to find your answers. They do not call the news TV programming for nothing.

Chapter 29

Conceptual Myth #7: Public Health Policy Is the Best Policy

Governments at all levels and in most countries around the world have adopted public health policies and guidelines that affect everything from drinking water sanitation and recommended vaccinations to food and nutrition support for the poor and public sanitation. We all want clean drinking water. We want proper disposal of trash and medical waste. We do not want factories and industrial plants dumping their chemical waste into our oceans, lakes and streams. These protections, most would agree, are positive. But these benefits are not the real substance of the discussion. The real issues are subtle and nearly invisible to all but those who have taken time to research the story.

For many, the idea that public health policy would be promulgated for anything except but the best interests of the people they purportedly serve is inconceivable. Yet there is a dilemma. We are also faced with a well-established and widely accepted public dogma that:

1) there are too many people on the planet;
2) this number of people is not sustainable;
3) resources, including food and clean water, are scarce and becoming more so;
4) we are consuming ourselves into a crisis;

5) something must be done to reduce the world's alleged overpopulation crisis; and
6) public assistance and Social Security–type programs will be unable to meet the demands of retirees.

Have you heard this? Do *you* believe this? Governments and large multinational corporations around the world have adopted these tenets as well, whether they are true or not. These issues and their potential solutions have been the subject of research and discussion at think tanks for decades. You only have to research the archives of the Rockefeller or Carnegie Foundations to see just how far back these ideas have been discussed.

So, if these principles are the *open* position of governments, large corporations and perhaps even you, why would public health policy support measures that extend life span, increase fertility, cure disease and promote optimal health? Why would governments want *more* people living longer, consuming more food, drinking more fresh water, using dwindling energy resources, accessing increasingly expensive medical and social services, relying on public assistance and drawing from Social Security–type programs than already do? Which policy do you think they follow? Do you believe they have your best interests in mind? What if public health policy was actually designed around what is best for government and the System, rather than you? Is there a rational basis for even asking these questions? I leave that for you to decide as you read along.

There are many deeper issues behind each of the questions articulated above and which have been the subject of research and discussion by others. It is beyond the scope of this work to delve into the global population discussion. My intent in mentioning these questions is to bring the *possibility* of such a disparity to your conscious awareness so that you may explore the concept further. But let us take just two brief examples to lend credibility to the larger question. One interesting example arises from the swine flu scare of 2009. As increasingly dire predictions of a global pandemic dominated the media, governments around the world purchased millions of doses of swine flu vaccine for their populations. But just as quickly, concerns about the safety of the yet untested and hastily approved H1N1 vaccine emerged, and acceptance by the public was generally poor. In Germany, the publication *Der Spiegel* reported that the German public was to be offered the GlaxoSmithKline vaccine Pandemrix, which contained a new adjuvant (a substance that amplifies the immune response)and mercury as the preservative. However, the German military and ranking government officials were to receive a special *clean* vaccine, Celvapan, which did not contain the powerful adjuvant or the mercury preservative. Why the double standard? Doesn't the fact that two different vaccines were produced validate the concern about the vaccine offered to the public? How would this information have affected your choice to accept the swine flu shot?

Let's look at another example, again related to vaccines. In a report issued in 2007, author F. William Engdahl describes the campaign launched in the 1990's by the UN's World Health Organization (WHO) to vaccinate women in Nicaragua, Mexico and the Philippines against tetanus – an illness that can arise from puncture wounds, such as stepping on a rusty nail. He points out that only women between the ages of 15 and 45 were targeted to receive the vaccine, although presumably men and boys had the same risk of stepping on a rusty nail, if not more so. This "anomaly" in the program caught the attention of a Roman Catholic lay organization, Comite Pro Vida de Mexico, who became suspicious and collected vaccine samples for testing. Engdahl then states:

> The tests revealed that the Tetanus vaccine being spread by the WHO only to women of child-bearing age contained human Chorionic Gonadotrophin or hCG, a natural hormone which when combined with a tetanus toxoid carrier stimulated antibodies rendering a woman incapable of maintaining a pregnancy. None of the women vaccinated were told.
>
> It later came out that the Rockefeller Foundation along with the Rockefeller's Population Council, the World Bank (home

to CGIAR), and the United States' National Institutes of Health had been involved in a 20-year-long project begun in 1972 to develop the concealed abortion vaccine with a tetanus carrier for WHO.

Additional reports indicate that in 1996, the Philippine Medical Association conducted its own research on behalf of the Philippine Department of Health and found that nine of the 47 vaccine samples tested positive for hCG. Similar findings were found in the Nicaragua and Mexico vaccines. This program affected 3 to 4 million women.

Whether you are willing to accept such health policies at face value will depend partly on your ability to access alternative information sources and your inclination to merely rely on government policies and, ultimately, the influences that operate through them. Please note the important distinction: the question is of blind trust in a *policy* of government, not of being "pro" or "anti" government. In fact, I expect that a more open and honest discussion about these policies would generate greater trust and cooperation between the citizenry and government. But until that time, it is important to remember that the people who largely control and run the governments around the world (not the elected faces shown on television) are a private lot who work together for *their* common goals and to promote *their* self-interests. This is really no secret; it is just not well publicized. Benjamin Disraeli, one of the great British politicians of the 19th Century who served twice as Prime Minister of England said, "The world is governed by very different personages from what is imagined by those who are not behind the scenes." US President Franklin Roosevelt has this to say in November 1933: "The real truth of the matter is, as you and I know, that a financial element in the larger centers has owned the government since the days of Andrew Jackson."

This self-appointed elite maintains vast cross-connections with governments, large corporations and international agencies. Just the cross-connections between the FDA and genetic engineering giant Monsanto would raise anyone's eyebrows. As many have said, it is a revolving door between FDA and the giant corporations such as Monsanto. However, these connections frequently remain unnoticed due to the manufactured paradigms of left versus right, Republican versus Democrat or conservative versus liberal which are sufficiently distracting to keep one's attention off the larger issues. But a growing number of people are beginning to see such labels as meaningless given that both political parties in the US, and probably the major political parties in many countries around the world, are financed and controlled by the same powerful interests. Whether we are talking about George Soros, Bill Gates, groups like *Media Matters*, the Rockefeller family or others, we are speaking about the true forces that guide and define public policy, including health policy. You only have to read books such as Professor Carroll Quigley's *Tragedy and Hope* to understand how this works.

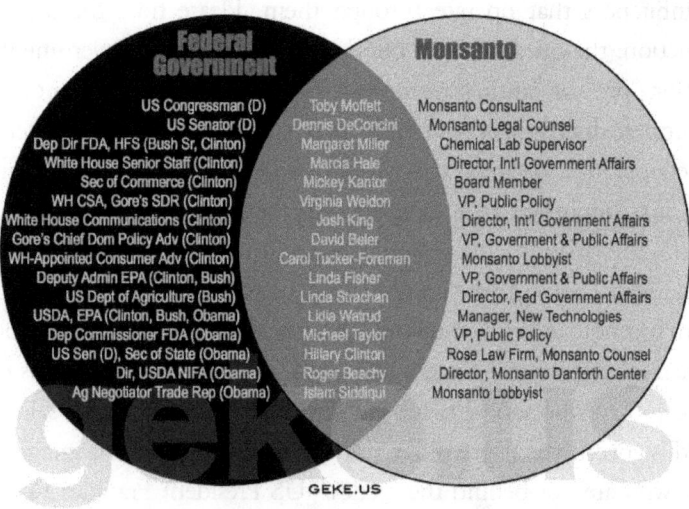

Figure 5: The Revolving Door between the US Federal Government and Monsanto. (Used with permission, http://geke.us)

Public health policy represents the *government's* recommendations for vaccinations, dealing with infectious diseases, sanitation and, in some countries, what you can and cannot say about how a food, plant, herb or nutritional compound might affect your health. In the US, the Food and Drug Administration (FDA) has assumed this authority. There, the FDA acts as the sole arbiter of what health claims any person or company can make about any substance, food, herb, liquid, energy device or any other object or substance that claims to prevent, treat, mitigate or cure any disease or infirmity. Whether you can provide independent scientific studies to support your claim is not sufficient justification for making a claim. The FDA must *agree* a claim is true for in order for it to be considered "true", at least in the US.

> "The American public does not have the knowledge to make wise health care decisions. The FDA is the arbiter of truth. Trust us. We will tell you what's good for you." – David Kessler, Commissioner FDA, 1998

Let's look at two examples of policy. In some countries, you may find an official policy position on preventing heart disease. That policy might sound something like, "Eat a low-fat, low-cholesterol diet, exercise and see your doctor". Although this is an easy message to convey to patients within the confines of a 15-minute medical appointment, the research shows that eating a low-fat, low-cholesterol diet will not produce the desired results, even if we assume that cholesterol is a *cause* of heart disease, which it is not. But of course, when diet fails (and this diet will fail), there are always drugs waiting in the wings! What about osteoporosis? The official policy might go something like this: "Exercise, eat a diet high in dairy products and other calcium-rich foods and see your doctor". Despite the cross-cultural studies that show high dairy intake is not associated with healthier bones, and despite the failure to recognize the importance of magnesium, potassium, boron, zinc, inflammation, insulin resistance, acid-blocker medications and a host of other critical factors in bone health, this simple and misleading message is still given to patients. Of course, when diet fails (and this diet will fail), there are drugs waiting in the wings again! Years ago I met with a woman who was diabetic and newly prescribed injectable insulin to help control her glucose levels. Diet alone had failed to adequately control her diabetes. Her physician had addressed the "nutrition part" by handing her a preprinted dietary sheet instructing her how to eat. The recommended diet was a high-carbohydrate, high-glycemic diet, front-loaded with carbohydrates in the morning. In the lower right corner of the page was the logo for the company who produced this convenient handout, which was the same drug company who produced the insulin. So why was she seeing me? Well, the diet was not working, and she was requiring more and more insulin to maintain her glucose levels!

For a number of people, especially those within the medical system, the FDA is regarded as a valuable protector of the public health through the regulation of drugs, inspection of food and so forth. Others regard the FDA as little more than a lobby for Big Pharma and a protector of conventional thinking in conventional medicine and the primary obstacle to genuine progress in all disciplines of medicine. Curiously, the FDA regards the drug companies that it is supposed to regulate as its "clients", not the American people.

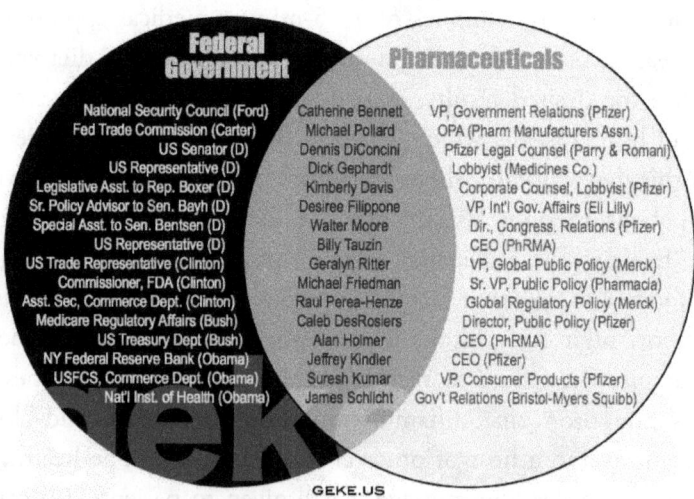

Figure 6: The Revolving Door between the US Government and Big Pharma (Used with permission, http://geke.us)

Your confidence in public health policy is partly based on your belief about the ethics (or lack thereof) of government. Does whatever government you live under tend to act in an ethical, moral manner? On what evidence do you base that belief? Does it serve the interests of the people or the interests of the elite who run the government? How far should government be allowed to go to force people to accept choices that they do not want or which violate their conscience? Should compulsory medical treatment be considered a legitimate authority of government?

Why is it that *government* is the force pushing for:

- Vaccines, whether you want them or not;
- Widespread use of GMO foods often without labeling or identification, despite all the consistent adverse health effects in all animal studies;
- Compulsory fluoridation of municipal water systems or table salt, even if the updated science demonstrates that it adversely impacts thyroid and bone health, damages the brain and lowers IQ, while it does not reduce tooth decay when taken systemically;
- The elimination of all sources of farm-fresh raw milk and raw dairy foods on the grounds that they are dangerous, even though the Queen and Royal family in England have it specially delivered to them and anyone can purchase it in vending machines in France;
- Enforcement of a policy that denies you a choice in how you treat your cancer, beyond the usual chemo, radiation or surgery; and
- Increased restriction and regulation of nutritional supplements (in the US, EU and Australia) when regulated drugs admittedly kill 106,000 Americans each year, and nutritional supplements (according to the US Poison Control Center) are alleged to have contributed to only 11 deaths in 26 years (although later analysis revealed that number to be zero).

Why is the push for these things *not* coming from the people? Why, when surveyed, do people overwhelmingly want *choice*, and not compulsion? Why does the government always resort to compulsion? Why is it that people must campaign *against* an agenda they did not initiate and do not want? Who is serving whom?

Governments are composed of people. As with all non-homogeneous groups, some people behave ethically and function within their authorized authority, and some do not. Throughout history, governments have done some pretty horrific things to their own people and to outsiders under the justification of war and even when at peace. Most ethical and moral people have a difficult time comprehending, even briefly, the mindset of those people who are capable of doing unspeakable things to their fellow humans, but there are many examples to point to in the 20th Century. Because these actions are beyond *our* comprehension, we tend to take a dangerous leap and conclude that it is also beyond the comprehension of everyone else, too. Sadly, such is not the case, and many honest, upstanding and civilized people have died as a result of not understanding the gravity of their circumstances until it was too late. When discovered, Truth has a way of changing things, sometimes dramatically.

How would you feel if you came to know that the government you now live under had conducted undisclosed experiments on its citizens or the citizens of other countries? If such a fact were true, how would it alter your sense of trust? Would you tend to view the government's health policies a bit differently? Would you even think to ask such a question? Why? Why not? Did you ever research that question? Why do we assume that because *we* would never do inhumane things, then no one else would ever do such things either?

When looking over the hundred years we call the 20th Century, what was the overall number-one killer of people on the planet? AIDS? Terrorism? Yellow fever? Cancer? Malnutrition? Plague? Snake bites?

According to the research of Professor Rudolph. J. Rummel, professor emeritus at the University of Hawaii, the number-one cause of death was, surprisingly, "democide". This topic has been extensively researched, and a number of works have been published.

The Wikipedia definition of "Democide" is:

> ...the murder of any person or people by a government, including genocide, politicide, and mass murder. Democide is not necessarily the elimination of entire cultural groups but rather groups within the country that the government feels need to be eradicated for political reasons and due to claimed future threats.
> [Note: Deaths on the battlefield are expressly *not* included in the term.]

As with most people, when I first heard this, I found it quite difficult to believe. Surely, something that *big*, that profound would be more widely known. The concept of a government killing people is deeply disturbing, and I suspect that for some readers, this segment of our discussion will generate a very high level of discomfort. Many people have never thought to investigate these and other important issues that critically affect where and how we place our trust. How many people have taken the time to do their homework on the safety of fluoride in drinking water? How many people have taken the time to verify how much mercury is actually in the annual flu shot or the neurological studies linking it to brain inflammation? How many people will take the time to understand the risks posed by GMO foods before passively accepting them into their diet?

Many educated people around the world, including perhaps the majority of Americans, have ever heard of Project MKUltra, the Tuskegee experiment, the experiments feeding radioactive oatmeal to retarded children in Massachusetts, the syphilis study conducted in Guatemala, the government-funded development of "spermicidal corn" or any of the dozens of documented examples from the last hundred years. Have you heard of these examples? Why not? If these examples are true, why did the media not cover these important stories? Where is the investigative journalism purportedly being conducted on your behalf? Where is the intellectual integrity? Where is the humanity? Wouldn't such a story be a worthy of some journalistic award? A Pulitzer Prize, perhaps? No, there is just silence, and if you bring any of these topics up, most people will experience such intense cognitive dissonance that their minds will close and they will scurry away. The truth can certainly make us uncomfortable. It can challenge authority. It can shatter our comfortable myths. But it also liberates us! As George Orwell so cogently stated: "In a time of universal deceit, telling the truth is a revolutionary act".

What about cancer? What if you or someone you loved was dealing with cancer and searching for a viable alternative to conventional treatment? How many people have heard of the alternative treatments pioneered by innovative medical doctors Max Gerson, Nicholas Gonzales or Stanislaw R. Burzynski? Would you prefer to have a choice? How difficult would it be for you to access such treatment?

What about the fluoride story? Is the fluoride added to the water supply really effective in preventing tooth decay? What about the studies linking fluoride exposure to lowered IQ, thyroid disease, bone fragility, kidney problems, glucose intolerance and even cancer? Why is there a warning on fluoride-containing toothpaste tubes alerting parents to call the poison control center if their child swallows the toothpaste on their toothbrush? Do you recall our earlier discussion of how this highly toxic substance was marketed as "beneficial"? Are you using fluoride toothpaste based on outdated "facts" and presumptions? There are questions and more questions, but the answers are there!

No doubt, these are some of the more perplexing questions we have raised thus far, and they are *not* raised to generate unfounded fear or suspicion, nor as an attempt to vilify any society or institution. From a personal perspective, our exposure to radically new information can feel a bit overwhelming at times. It is during these times that we can recall the reassuring words of Mahatma Gandhi when he addressed these very same issues:

> "When I despair, I remember that all through history the ways of truth and love have always won. There have been tyrants, and murderers, and for a time they can seem invincible, but in the end they always fall. Think of it—always."

And thus, the questions outlined here are raised to help us recalibrate our perceptions and speak to the many reasons why we need to redirect our energies, faith, trust and power back to ourselves and our local communities, where we can most effectively direct it to positive use. There is no safer, more effective repository of the responsibility for your health and that of your family than in *your* hands. To be sure, there will be times when you need to engage the services of a medical or other health professional. But when you do your homework and accept that the final authority rests with you, those practitioners whose judgment and abilities you decide to trust are likely to produce a better clinical outcome.

Chapter 30

Conceptual Myth #8: False Evidence Appearing Real (F.E.A.R.)

"He who fears he shall suffer, already suffers what he fears." – Montaigne

Fear is one of the most powerful, primitive emotions we can experience. Fear may save our life or paralyze us, depending on the source. Either way, fear alters our physiology to prepare us to run or fight. In a fearful state, our cognitive thinking capacity is diminished, and we resort to more primal reflex actions than conscious, planned responses.

Some fears are rational, while others are quite irrational. If you were to walk around all day wringing your hands in desperate anxiety about being killed by a falling meteorite, I dare say most people would judge that fear to be unwarranted. What are the odds of that really occurring? According to the US National Safety Council, the chance of dying from an asteroid impact is between 1 in 200,000 and 1 in 500,000. Contrast that with a 1 in 5 lifetime chance of dying of heart disease or 1 in 100 lifetime chance of dying in a car accident. The odds of being struck by lightning are 1 in 576,000. Is the fear of being killed by a falling asteroid justified? You decide. But whether you feel that such a fear is "justified" or "rational" or not, there is little you can do about to protect yourself, unless you wish to live deep underground in a bunker, and even that would only protect against a small asteroid!

If you make the mistake of turning on the television and tuning into the news provided by the media, you will be bombarded with messages about the latest war, bombing or uprising and a promotional campaign for the latest battle against the purported bad guys. And don't forget the corollary message that no one is safe and no one can be trusted. You can see what this belief has done to air travel. You are expected to buy into the media's information on the risks of terrorism as factual because the newscasters tell you so. How much fear is warranted? According to the National Safety Council, you are eight times more likely to be killed by a police officer than a terrorist. You are nine times more likely to choke to death on your own vomit than be killed by a terrorist. In fact, more Americans have been killed by bee stings or falling televisions than by terrorists. Being in a state of fear alters your thinking and decisions, whether your fear concerns terrorism or worry about being killed by a falling asteroid. Sometimes you can disengage fear with compelling truth. You can also disengage fear by trusting yourself, your intuition, your higher consciousness and your personal life path. As you reduce your level of fear, you can more easily access your intuition and inspiration from within.

For those who have grown up with fearful parents or other adult figures, you may have modeled that behavior as *your* response to life. Specific or non-specific chronic fears may also arise from the experiences and traumas that we can have in the course of our lives. There are a number of newer therapeutic methods that have shown great promise in releasing the patterns of fear and phobias. I discuss them in the last section of this book and invite anyone who is held captive by torments of the mind and irrational fears of what might be to explore these methods.

Fearing what might happen in life is nothing unusual. Even satirist Mark Twain acknowledged the fear of what could be, saying, "I am an old man and have known a great many troubles, but most of them never happened."

The experience of fear alters our perceptions, and we begin to view life from a perspective of survival and then make decisions accordingly. Fear about survival is the most basic of human emotions; it includes elements of scarcity, lack and limitation. People who can be maintained in a fearful state are usually more easily managed and controlled.

John Leach of Lancaster, England is one of the leading experts in survival psychology and why people do or do not survive in a crisis. His work is quoted by military survival training schools around the world, and he teaches British forces how to survive in almost any circumstance. Leach's research has lead to the Theory of 10-80-10, which provides valuable insight into how people handle crises in life.

Leach's research found that approximately 10 percent of the population responds to a crisis with relative calm and a rational state of mind. These people tend to be able to pull themselves together quickly, make a rational assessment of the situation, establish priorities, create a plan and take action with clarity and focus. These are the kind of people you want around you in a crisis. Or, better yet, strive to be one of these people in a crisis!

The "80" stands for the vast majority of people—the 80 percent—who when suddenly faced with a crisis will feel stunned and bewildered and experience impaired reasoning and thinking capabilities. In this state, people are more likely to stare straight ahead, barely hearing the people around them. They become lethargic and will feel their heart racing along with a queasy, sick feeling. Some people may call this experience "brain-lock" or "brain-freeze". Although this incapacitating sensation is temporary, it can delay important actions that ensure survival. These people may tend to be in shock and prefer to wait for others or the authorities to tell them what to do.

The last group of people—that last 10 percent—are the ones you do not want to have around you in any bona fide emergency. These are the people who lose control and freak out. Their resulting behavior is frequently counterproductive to their own survival and makes the situation worse.

For any of us, predicting how we might react in a true crisis is reasonably difficult. Whether you will become part of the solution, the group waiting for a solution or that last group working against a solution is an unknown for most. However, with practice and by adopting a preparedness attitude, anyone can increase their likelihood of joining the Top 10 Percent that is capable of helping yourself and perhaps others to survive. Whether the crisis comes in the form of a capsizing boat or a personal experience, the odds are that most of us will have some first-hand experience with crisis. An excellent book on this topic is *The Survivors Club* by Ben Sherwood.

For many people, dealing with fear is an important component in the quest for healthy, balanced living. By dissipating groundless fears or seeing through all other fears, we may access our higher cognitive faculties and escape the damaging effects incurred by perpetually bathing our cells in a sea of stress hormones as we discussed in Chapter 13.

The Challenge of Being Positive

Finding a balance point between being positive and seeing the negative is a challenge for most people emerging into Consciousness, especially those souls who are self-described as sensitive types. You know who you are. We believe that focusing on the positive elements of our life and our future has the ability to attract more positive people, events and circumstances into our lives. Such practices do appear to work for many people, but whether the outcome is a product of conscious or subconscious thoughts and beliefs is not always clear.

The example I would like to offer to illustrate this point is recalled from my many years sailing off the coast of Maine in the United States. Maine waters are beautiful to sail and explore. Whales, ospreys, eagles, seals and some incredible scenery are part of the magic of sailing Downeast. (For readers who may not know, "Downeast" is a regional term that refers to the ocean waters of mid to northern Maine.) But as any sailor knows, Maine waters are challenging. There are significant tides and currents, rapidly changing weather conditions, the notorious Maine fog, rocks and underwater ledges and, of course, lobster pots everywhere! Chatting dockside with seasoned sailors will undoubtedly recall stories of sailors hitting submerged rocks, breaking keels and even sinking. All told, there are enough stories to give the sober sailor a healthy respect for the environment.

When sailing in Maine, it was pretty much a necessity to watch for breaking water, rocks, ledges and other hazards that might make for a really bad day. Standing at the helm, I had a charted course to follow, but I was constantly scanning the waters ahead and around me for potential hazards. Could we rightly say that I was "being negative" by "looking for" the submerged rocks, underwater ledges and lobster pots? If my sole focus was the boat's course (a more positive perspective), and I never looked for the problems (the negative perspective), then I might have risked making it safely to my destination? Sometimes it is prudent to look for the problem in order to protect and achieve the positive goal. Looking for the problem does not mean we have to dwell on the problem. We just have to acknowledge it and continue to move along our path.

Chapter 31

Conceptual Myth #9: You Can Save Time and Money

Our concept of time is an interesting one. If you ask most people in Westernized cultures about time, you will hear at least two fairly consistent themes: 1) that they don't have enough time, and 2) that time moves in one direction. We refer to the latter concept all the time when speaking of "moving forward" or "looking back". And because we think of time as an arrow flying in one direction, we can only hope to slow down or speed up its flight. To date, I do not know of anyone who has accomplished such a feat, but everyone would like to know how to do so.

We also speak of time as a commodity. We try to work several tasks at once to "save" time. We clear our schedule so we can "spend" time with the family. We rearrange when we will do things to try to "buy" time. When we walk the dog, we "take" time. When we engage in meaningless activity waiting for something we see as more valuable, we try to "kill" time. Of course, if we do not "take" time, then how can we ever "have" time? Time does not even seem to be consistent. When you are doing something with someone you love, time "flies". According to Jimmy Buffett, when you are waiting for a flight in the San Juan airport, "five minutes feels like a day".

In other cultures, particularly in South American and shamanic-based peoples, time is conceptualized more like an unfolding than an arrow. The metaphor I have heard most often used here is that of a rose blossoming and opening. Author Gregg Braden discusses this concept of time in great detail in his book *Fractal Time,* and the notion that time exists in both waves and in cycles is in contradistinction to the concept of the unidirectional linear time line. But regardless of how you conceptualize time, how we manage our time seems to be a universal challenge.

One of the most common complaints that I hear from people who have chosen to rebuild or enhance their health via natural principles is that doing so *takes time*. It takes more time to read the labels, shop for fresh produce, prepare healthy meals and plan ahead for lunch or other meals when the schedule hits a snag. This assessment is correct on all counts. Choosing natural foods does take time, awareness and purpose. But the commitment of our time is an unnecessary obstacle created by both our beliefs and perceptions. Brain research tells us that our perception of time varies by the physiological state we are in. Not surprisingly, our sense of time is altered by stress hormones. When the brain is awash in cortisol, one of our primary stress hormones, we commonly experience a sense that there is not enough time. Even if we were to analyze the situation objectively and demonstrate the lack of time to be untrue, the feeling that we are lacking sufficient time persists, and we make decisions based on that distorted perception. Leonardo Da Vinci said that "Time stays long enough for anyone who will use it".

In some respects, how people handle the time versus health equation is analogous to how they would approach their future financial goals, even though such a link is rarely made. In the financial world, we are admonished to plan for the future by diverting a portion of current earnings toward a future time in the expectation that we will have it to rely upon later in life. If you asked a 22 year old what sort of financial health they would like to experience when they are 65, you might hear them say that they "hope" to be well-off, or they "hope" to have enough money to travel or they "hope" to have a nice home. But "hoping" does not constitute a plan. In the same way, if you ask someone what kind of health they would like to enjoy when they reach 70, they might answer, "I hope I don't have arthritis", "I hope I don't get cancer" or "I hope I don't have diabetes". Hope is a good start, but not a plan.

In matters of both physical and emotional health, thinking of time as a commodity to be invested can be very useful. The state of health and well-being you hope to have when you are 70 will tend to be, to a certain degree, the product of your investment all along the way. Taking time *earlier* and investing it into your personal health or your family's health pays dividends *later* in life when you want it or need it. Perhaps this is the basis for author Alice Bloch's perspective when she said: "We say we waste time, but that is impossible. We waste ourselves."

Temptations will come. Many of the behaviors, foods, beverages and other products that contribute to poor health and disease are marketed using the illusion of "saving time" and your belief that you can do so by purchasing them. Whether you are traveling on the highway, flying to a destination or simply living your busy day-to-day at home, if you have not given advanced thought to meals, then you are likely to be at the mercy of so-called fast food. As everyone now knows, fast foods are typically highly processed foods, infused with various chemicals and preservatives to prolong shelf life, retard spoilage and excite the taste buds. These food options are prepared at an undisclosed location from the cheapest quality ingredients in an effort to create the largest profit for the seller. What a deal!

Grabbing a burger for lunch on the road or a microwaved rubber egg sandwich in lieu of a healthy breakfast at home are habits that *may* seem justified at the moment, but really only etch away our resilience and diminish our energy. We have to ask ourselves, what was the benefit we received in this deal? Did I save time? How many minutes? Ten? Fifteen? The point of this discussion is not to judge those rare situations that you could not have possibly foreseen, such as unexpectedly having to spend time in a waiting room at a hospital waiting to hear how a loved one is doing in the ER. Our day-to-day habits are the concern and make the difference.

In the current commerce-is-everything society, you will always be enticed to trade in your health for sake of convenience. We face this choice consciously or unconsciously. If you choose to take the bait and buy fast foods in an attempt to save time today, what do you think the outcome will likely be tomorrow? A cancer? Heart disease? Type II diabetes? Obesity? Arthritis? Stroke? These and many other disease states have their genesis in diet and nutrition.

Fast forward 40 years. Suppose you spent all those years "saving time" and "saving money" by eating grab-and-go fast foods and now you face a diagnosis of heart disease. Are you surprised? Dealing with the various diagnostic tests, angiograms, cardiac catheterizations, visits to specialists, trips to the pharmacy, hospital stays, waiting for radiologists and so on now all consume time and money. If you were able to do the math, I would bet that dealing with your poor health later in life would consume all that time and money you *thought you saved* years before, and then some. What is even worse is that you probably do not even enjoy the time you are currently living. As they say, "payback's a bitch". Maybe you saved some money for travel, but now you cannot walk very far without chest pain or leg cramps. The fistful of drugs you have to take each day contributes a raft of additional symptoms. Or you had a stroke, and your physical mobility and dexterity are limited. Turns out that fast foods were not a very good investment. All that time we thought we *saved* is now paid back with interest, *high interest*. The illusion of saving time is another marketing image fostered by Big

Agra, Big Pharma and Big Business in concert with Big Government. It is their gain and your loss, cloaked under the illusion of saving time.

Choosing to invest your time *now* in a way that produces benefits and dividends for *you* both now and in the future is the only sane way to go. There is no short cut or miracle cure that will undo years of self-delusion and self-abuse endured for the sake of your schedule. Yes, you are trying to make a living, but are you really just making a killing—of yourself? This question brings us to a sobering observation. We come to the realization, sometimes too late, that we are all involuntarily enrolled in a system and a society that rewards committed self-destruction. If you ever worked for a major corporation, you understand how they value you. The good news is that once you are aware of this, you can choose to opt out. How? Doing so is actually simple. You opt out one day at a time, by each healthy meal you take the time to eat, with each evening that you go to bed at a healthy time and by every occasion you take time to go for a walk. You remind yourself that the time you take to eat a healthy lunch, take a vacation or rest on a Saturday afternoon is time *invested*, not lost. You make and affirm that decision to invest in *you* each day, every day and all day.

Chapter 32

Conceptual Myth #10: Modern Medicine IS Medicine

Modern medicine and the prevailing medical industry would like you to believe that *it* is the only legitimate form of medicine and that it is based on sound science and objective research. As pointed out in Myth #4, there is more to that story than meets the eye. So how did this belief get started?

Historically, the general term "medicine" included a diverse array of different and competing philosophies, disciplines and practices. Prior to 1910, people could choose between physicians practicing within any number of competing schools of thought. From the early to mid-1800s, you had the option of seeing homeopathic physicians. These healers followed the principles of Samuel Hannahman, MD, who utilized potent homeopathic "micro-doses" known as "remedies" to treat both acute and chronic conditions. Homeopathy is based on the principle known as "The Law of Similars" or "like cures like." Meanwhile, osteopathic physicians offered treatment and preventive medicine through osteopathic manipulation and associated practices. Chiropractic appeared around 1896 and gradually trained practitioners in chiropractic manipulation. Around the turn of the century, naturopathy appeared as an offshoot of the European Nature Cure movement. And, of course, herbalists have been around since time began, employing botanical extracts, tinctures and poultices for any number of conditions. The School of Natural Hygiene also had its adherents and practitioners. And, there was the school of medicine referred to as allopathic medicine (also known then as heroic medicine). The term "heroic medicine" referred to the practice of using large doses of pharmacologically active agents or physical interventions to treat and suppress symptoms or the processes of disease. This approach is what we know today as "modern medicine" or "conventional medicine".

In the mid- to late 1800s in the US, opiate compounds were readily available and legally sold over the counter to treat coughs, tuberculosis and pain. With names such as Ayer's Cherry Pectoral, Mrs. Winslow's Soothing Syrup, McMunn's Elixir of Opium and Dover's Powder, pain could now be controlled in a way not previously available. Wealthy business tycoons, such as the Rockefellers and the Carnegies, saw a profitable future in drugs and invested heavily in their development and promotion. Ironically, these and other wealthy families of the day chose to be treated by homeopathic physicians, not allopathic physicians, a trend that continues today.

In 1908, the newly formed Council on Medical Education within the AMA (American Medical Association) asked the Carnegie Foundation for the Advancement of Teaching to survey the American medical schools of the time in the hopes of promoting their Continuing Education agenda. The Carnegie Foundation agreed and hired Abraham Flexner to conduct the survey. It took Flexner five years to complete his survey of all 155 medical schools. In 1910, the "Flexner Report" was published. This report was the beginning of the end for almost all of the non-heroic medical schools. Those medical schools that were pharmaceutical-based received massive financial investment from the Rockefeller and Carnegie families, who were already heavily invested in the newly developing pharmaceutical industry. Those medical schools that were not pharmaceutical-based were denied such support. Thus, a hugely uneven and unequal playing field was created between pharmaceutical-based medicine and all the others schools of medicine. Between 1910 and 1935, more than half of all American medical schools either closed or merged. To maintain accreditation, the remaining medical schools that taught homeopathic medicine, chiropractic, osteopathic medicine or naturopathic medicine had to cease doing so or close their doors. Gradually, state medical boards adopted the recommendations of the Flexner Report, which included a recommendation that no new medical school could open without permission of the state and that the state branch of the American Medical Association would have oversight of all allopathic medical schools within that state. Thus, the AMA achieved dominance and ultimately political and legislative control over the entire field of medicine. This authority was not based on superior science or superior results, but as a result of massive financial investment from the Carnegie and Rockefeller families to bolster the growth of the pharmaceutical industry in which they were so heavily invested. Likewise, modern medicine is where it is today not because of superior results or a superior philosophy but because of financial dominance protected by legislative force. Had a level playing field been protected, we might enjoy the best of all the medical modalities with an improvement in the human condition.

When we speak of "medicine" in the broad, generic sense of the term, we can include all other forms of medicine not included within the current monopoly structure. Allopathic medicine, just like naturopathic medicine and herbal medicine, is first a philosophy of medicine, and each philosophy uses tools and techniques to express the principles of that philosophy. Modern allopathic medicine uses some science to support its philosophy and treatment approach to disease. But it would be incorrect to state that modern medicine *is* science to the exclusion of all other forms of medicine. Science is the search for Truth. According to Dictionary.com it can be characterized as:

- systematic knowledge of the physical or material world gained through observation and experimentation;
- any of the branches of natural or physical science;
- systematized knowledge in general; and
- knowledge, as of facts or principles; knowledge gained by systematic study.

Modern medicine relies on a type of science referred to as reductionism. Reductionism is a perspective that presumes and believes that you can know a complex "thing" by understanding all of its parts and that the whole is nothing more than the sum of its parts. From this perspective, you, as a complex living and breathing being, can be understood thoroughly if we could just find a way to break everything down into smaller and smaller bits. Reductionism is the opposite of holism (holistic). It is a micromanager's dream!

Other perspectives within the field of science include: observational science, empirical science, inductive science, deductive science and more. So, if one conducted a research project to test whether a homeopathic remedy was effective on a particular condition, one could scientifically conclude that it was effective or ineffective even if one did not understand the mechanism of how it worked. This is the "knowledge of the physical or material world gained through observation and experimentation" part of the definition of science, but it is not the science of reductionism. Readers may be surprised to learn that for many drugs actively and routinely prescribed today, it is not truly known how they work, although the drug company does provide a theory for how researchers *think* the drug works. Understanding the mechanism for how a thing works is not a prerequisite for pronouncing something as "scientific" or "legitimate" or not. Most people flip their light-switch to turn on a light without understanding the mechanism of where and how that power is created, regulated, metered and delivered to the wire in their home. We do not necessarily need to know. The same is true with homeopathy, energy healing, herbal medicine and other approaches to healthcare. We may not have the foggiest idea how they work, and the tendency to accept or reject them is based not on understanding, but familiarity. We are familiar with drug medicine, even if we do not necessarily want to rely upon it. But if we are unfamiliar with energy healing or the principles of homeopathy, we will most likely question its legitimacy. Healthy skepticism is good; it can save us from those dishonest schemes and products that offer nothing but the illusion of hope. But if we use these criteria to examine the statistics and years of data compiled about modern medicine, then how would we judge the legitimacy of the current medical system? Outside of the recognized benefits in emergency and acute care situations, where are the benefits in either treatment or prevention to stem the rising tsunami of chronic disease?

Witness people's reactions when a local hospital goes through a huge expansion in both the number of patients it can serve and the degree and complexity of medical services it can offer. The hospital and many in the community laud such an expansion as "progress". Certainly it is a testament to the economic success of medicine and of the hospital, but is it really progress? Why is the necessity to have more patient beds, more operating rooms, bigger rehab space, more physicians, more CT scanners, more MRI units and so on in order to treat more sick people viewed as progress? Why are there so many more sick people needing treatment? Might be more accurate to state that the need for a bigger hospital is really a hard-reality indicator that because more people are ill and more people need treatment, then modern medicine has ultimately failed to improve the health of the population? If all the millions of dollars poured into modern medicine translated into better health for the population, would we not need smaller hospitals? It does make one pause to reflect.

Chapter 33

Conceptual Myth #11: Choice and the Law of Causality

Whether we are speaking of the biological sciences or physics, our lives are governed by certain rules and principles that we refer to as the Laws of Nature. We all need oxygen, clean water, food, specific elements we call nutrients, sleep and so forth. We are governed by gravity and affected by both visible and invisible radiation that includes everything from visible light to the ionizing radiation of x-rays. When our cells are provided with quality raw materials, we can repair damage and produce new cells of excellent quality. Our biology responds to the presence or absence of stimuli, such as sound, vibration, heat, cold or pressure.

Our human biology is very much driven by cause and effect. Fortunately, we do not malfunction suddenly and for no reason. You do not suddenly vomit for no reason while driving your car. Your body will not produce excruciating pain in your left ankle unless there is a reason to attract your attention. To believe the contrary is to adopt a very unsettling view that your body does a poor job at self-regulation, is inherently stupid and may suddenly and mysteriously malfunction at any moment with no particular reason for such an experience. Such is not the case.

That being said, many people who end up in a state of chronic poor mental or physical health seem to have adopted the latter view. How can that be? Such an observation can only be made when we review how a person with chronic fatigue syndrome or fibromyalgia has lived or, more accurately, attempted to live over the preceding years. As many natural medicine practitioners have observed, there is a common theme of behavior and attitude—a psychology—among people diagnosed with these two conditions in particular. There are similar patterns of behavior, attitudes and beliefs in the diabetic. Because our attitudes and beliefs drive our behaviors, achieving true healing necessitates that we discover and modify the underlying perspectives that allowed for the creation of the symptoms. Falling short of doing so will produce partial and temporary amelioration of the symptoms with an eventual return to the same disabled state.

For everyone on the journey of healing, accepting responsibility for where they are and the actions that led them there is a huge and necessary step. Accepting responsibility is not about blaming. It about becoming aware of the cause-and-effect relationship that is always in play, accepting that it is so and being willing to change that which is not working toward our highest good. Here are some of the behaviors that represent the "cause" half of the "cause and effect" equation:

- Driving into the fast food drive-thru for a breakfast sandwich or bagel and coffee because you did not allow enough time to eat a healthy meal at home;
- Staying up until 2 AM each night to "get things done", violating your body's critical circadian rhythm and biological clock;
- Not drinking enough water because you do not want to have to urinate that frequently;

- Making food choices purely on the basis of taste or convenience without appreciating the health and nutritive impact of the food; and
- Relying on quick, processed foods because you did not plan ahead or allow enough time to prepare the meal.

These examples and hundreds more are elements of the Law of Causality. Whether you understand it, like it or even know it exists, it is the operating principle running in the background of all choices you make. It is what moves people toward illness and emotional distress and helps keep them locked in self-perpetuating cycles. The popular phrase "keep doing what you are doing and you will keep getting what you are getting" is another way of expressing this effect. The downside of the cause-and-effect cycle may be engaged through either ignorance or arrogance.

Ignorance is easy to understand. You just did not understand or appreciate that what you eat, think, drink, read, watch and believe all affect your physical and emotional state. While it may be difficult to comprehend how anyone could have total ignorance of what appears to be a common-sense principle, it nevertheless remains beyond the awareness of some people. The arrogance issue is a more subtle perspective that arises from a desire or belief that you can live life based on the desires of the mind and be immune to the consequences to the body.

Consider sleep as an example. In the case where people violate their chrono-biology by habitually going to bed at 1 AM or 2 AM, they have often rationalized that they are so-called night people and staying up late is normal for them. Not recognizing that they are part of nature, not separate from nature, and that the cycles of light and dark are key synchronizing signals for our biological clock, they deny themselves an important benefit of working *with* their natural biological rhythms. Failing to honor our innate rhythms creates not only immediate effects, but also ripple effects that permeate our entire physiology. This effect is demonstrated in studies that have shown that sleep deprivation is a risk factor for developing diabetes. This effect also explains why almost 99% of the clients I have seen who are dealing with some variant of chronic fatigue syndrome or fibromyalgia habitually go to bed well after midnight. Research suggests that eight hours of sleep acquired between 2 AM and 10 AM is not of the same restorative quality as eight hours of sleep from 9 PM to 5 AM. In countries where the clock is changed each spring and fall for Daylight Savings Time, most people can feel an internal disturbance similar to jet lag even though they did not go anywhere. Jet lag is a more obvious example of what happens when we are out of sync with the natural light/dark cycle. Instinctively, we all know this is true, but sometimes our mind has another agenda.

Rebellion and Bondage

For many people fully entrenched in the frenetic pace of modern living, daily life may feel a bit regimented or restrictive. Having little choice but to work five or more days each week to pay a host of monthly costs associated with modern living—the rent or mortgage, utilities, food, transportation, insurance and so on—it can begin to feel as if we are locked into a pattern of increasing rigidity and decreasing freedom. Feeling confined or without a sense of control, we often search for ways to reassert that diminished sense of freedom and exercise control. For many, there is no easier way to do so than through food.

Sometimes, in a desperate, emotional attempt to feel in control, we may say to ourselves, "I'll eat what I want, when I want" as an act of rebellion against the inflexible nature of our daily routine. In fact, we might even feel quite powerful deciding to eat what we shouldn't as part of our act of defiance, right? After all, you are taking control! You have decided, "I want that bowl of ice cream *now*. I don't care if it isn't good for me!" Whether this act arises from the child in us or the emotionally frustrated adult is a question I leave to the psychologists. Either way, food becomes our tool in our quest to reestablish a sense of control and freedom.

While we may experience short-term satisfaction in our acts of defiance and rebellion, our chronic disregard for the Laws of Nature and Causality brings consequences, such as poor physical or mental health or even a specific disease. Here again, nature is not without a sense of irony. Our freedom, then, lies in following the rules: the Laws of Nature. Yes, it seems like the ultimate oxymoron, doesn't it? How can following rules result in freedom? Actually, the concept is neither new nor complicated. When we *choose* to adhere to the natural principles that support good health, we are freed from the bondage of chronic illness. In this case, the seemingly paradoxical statements "our rebellion creates our bondage" and "there is freedom through following the rules" are both quite literally true. Understanding these rules is the first step, and exercising choice is the second step.

Recognizing the power of causality is a key principle in the quest to break free from the invisible chains that bind us to poor health and lowered vitality. Through awareness and recognition, we can change our thinking, our habits and our choices in order to create a new, healthier outcome. Cause and effect works both ways—toward bondage or toward freedom. It is always a choice, but not always a choice made consciously! However, *knowing* it is a choice now allows to you exercise that choice to your benefit anytime you are ready!

Recognizing and understanding the impact of the Conceptual Myths we have now discussed, is an important step in our journey toward better health. But our search for better health is intimately coupled to a search for truth for it is in the revelation of truth that we are empowered to make positive choices. Mahatma Gandhi once said it this way: "In the attitude of silence the soul finds the path in a clearer light, and what is elusive and deceptive resolves itself into crystal clearness. Our life is a long and arduous quest after Truth".

Part VI

Personal Emancipation: Reclaiming Your Power

> "Power is of two kinds. One is obtained by the fear of punishment and the other by acts of love. Power based on love is a thousand times more effective and permanent than the one derived from fear of punishment." – Mohandas K. Gandhi

The power we speak of in this section is the second kind of power that Gandhi refers to in the quote above: the kind of power from acts of love. Here we speak of acts of self-love, love of family, love of beauty, love of humanity and love of life. This love is intertwined with self-respect and respect for others and the gifts that they bring.

Chapter 34

Reclaiming Your Power

Reclaiming your personal power is accomplished through active steps, both positive and negative. Active positive steps are things that you consciously choose to do based on an understanding of their benefit, such as eating clean, organically-grown food, meditating each morning, getting into your far infrared sauna three times per week to lower your total body burden of toxins and so on. But perhaps the biggest gains you will make in regaining your power are by using the Word of Power in what is known as an apophatic process. "Apophatic" comes from the Greek root word *apophanai*, meaning to say "no". Relative to the many invitations you receive each day to surrender your power, privacy, health, hard-earned money and sanity, saying "no" is one of the most powerful words you can utter and stand upon. Lest you think this word's power is being a bit overstated, recall that in India Mahatma Gandhi brought the British Empire to its knees by using the power of "no". Exercising the power of "no" benefits not just you, but also it creates ripple effects to benefit those you care about and others you do not even know. This concept is not new and is echoed in the timeless words of Leonardo da Vinci: "Nothing strengthens authority so much as silence".

Every time you say "no", whether it is to the processed-food drive-thru beckoning to you on your way home from work, to the fear-driven flu shot hyped by your pharmacy or medical provider or to the antidepressant drug prescribed to mask the normal feeling of grief when a loved one dies, you not only spare yourself later consequences but also you retain authenticity and responsibility for your life experiences. You are honoring the principle of cause and effect and working it to *your* benefit rather than for the benefit of the System.

One of the most inspiring and majestic moments in contemporary film that exemplifies this principle unfolds toward the end of the first *Matrix* movie, where the hero Neo falls to the ground after being shot by Agent Smith and his colleagues. His love of Trinity restores him to life, and upon standing up to again face agent Smith, Neo holds up his hand and utters just one word with total conviction: the Word of Power, "no"! And that moment is the turning point in Neo's transformation as "The One". In reality, we are each "The One" in our own lives, and we each face the challenge of owning our power through belief in ourselves. Even if you are not particularly fond of futuristic sci-fi movies, you cannot miss the dramatic symbolism in *The Matrix* that speaks to these universal and powerful truths.

Reclaiming your personal power is a process of reversing the direction of flow and divesting it from those people, images, symbols, institutions and agencies that work to collect it. This process, therefore, is one of decentralization, with the ultimate localization back within you!

This process of decentralizing power back to you is one that you can practice daily. In fact, you will have many opportunities during a day to reclaim and retain your power, as you begin to notice how frequently, and often subtly, you are being enticed to surrender it. One of the easiest ways to begin this process is by opting out of the various offers, programs or technologies that draw power and information away from you as we will discuss in upcoming sections. As you and others begin to vest your power back to yourselves, it becomes easier for others to do so and eventually change society.

There may be a more powerful incentive to growth and change than illness. Illness can be the push that we need to re-examine our lives, what we were so busy doing before we became ill and how we are going to respond to the immediate challenge. Whether we have one of the many lifestyle diseases, such as Type II diabetes, or risk factors, such as elevated cholesterol or triglycerides, we can look past the symptoms and examine the underlying problems.

Chapter 35

Challenge Your Current Health Paradigm

"Nothing can stop the man with the right mental attitude from achieving his goal; nothing on earth can help the man with the wrong mental attitude." – Thomas Jefferson

If you have a health condition, or a specific, named disease, here are some questions that may help elucidate where you might be limited in your thinking or off in your perception:

- How do you view your condition or disease? Do you view it as a thing or as merely a name given to some condition or group of symptoms?

- Do you believe your condition is the result of random chance or poor genes? Do you feel like a victim?

- What habits, beliefs, emotions or traumas do you feel contributed to your illness or condition? Did your MS come on after a significant grief or loss? Is your fibromyalgia your body's way of setting boundaries that you could not set voluntarily?

- What does your illness do *for* you? Most chronic illness has a secondary benefit that we value but do not readily admit.

Is there a hidden benefit, such as getting more attention, avoiding certain major life questions or controlling those around you?

- Has anyone else *ever* experienced a full recovery or remission from the exact condition that you have? Even if the odds were 1 in 100,000, do you believe you can be that "1"?

- What will you *not* do or *not* change to experience a substantial improvement in your health? Why not? Why are those things non-negotiable?

- What attitudes or emotions do you feel have contributed to your condition? What attitudes or emotions are holding you back from recovery?

- Are you waiting for the latest drug or the newest treatment to come along and rescue you?

- Do you doubt your ability to research and explore other healing methods?

- Do you think you may have one or more "nocebo" beliefs that are sabotaging your health?

- Are you more comfortable delegating the responsibility for your life and your health to your physician, and are you willing to accept the consequences?

- Have all the treatments you have tried originated from within the same medical school of thought (such as allopathic medical)? Are you expecting a different outcome from each new treatment within the same medical model?

Not surprisingly, exploring the answers to these questions can help dissipate much of the power an illness may hold over us. A shift in our perception may allow us to see and pursue avenues we had not considered or even thought existed. That is not to suggest that once you discern the answers to the questions you will jump up magically cured; but it may be a critical step toward removing the obstacles that prevent your body from doing the healing it is innately designed to do. Shifting your perception may remove the distortion in your energy field that created the imbalance in the first place. Doing so just may lead you to new therapeutic techniques and methods that you would have dismissed previously as unrelated simply because you could not see the relationship. Know this: everything about you is connected! Everything! While ancient spiritual traditions have taught this concept for eons, the interconnectedness of everything has been recognized in the world of quantum physics for nearly a hundred years. As Nobel Prize winning physicist Max Planck once said:

> All matter originates and exists only by virtue of a force which brings the particle of an atom to vibration and holds this most minute solar system of the atom together. We must assume behind this force the existence of a conscious and intelligent mind. This mind is the matrix of all matter.

Chapter 36

Expanding Your Personal Power

"There is a power inside every human against which no earthly force is of the slightest consequence." – Neville Goddard

There is much you can do to increase your focus and thereby increase your power. A light bulb and a laser both emit light, but the photons emitted by the laser are focused ("coherent" is the proper term), making that light able to cut steel while light from the light bulb cannot. The changes you make are the result of your conscious intent to alter how you live, see reality, react to events and create your experiences. The point is, this is all driven by your conscious intent! And it is something we all practice on our journey.

If you have any condition other than robust, vital health, then you owe it to yourself to explore other methods to restore your health that you may not currently be using. Perhaps you are comfortable with clinical nutrition as a bona fide therapeutic approach. But on the other hand, you say you "don't believe" in homeopathy, or acupuncture, or energy healing, or "fill in the blank". When we exclude a choice that we do not understand simply because we do not understand it, we severely limit our potential for healing and for life. We may not blindly accept every notion or product pitched in our direction, but to blindly reject those therapies that have been around for decades, if not hundreds of years, is to volunteer to stay solidly inside the box. As Albert Einstein said, "The greatest form of ignorance is to reject something you know nothing about".

So, do not be afraid to push your thinking to new limits. To accomplish this, you do not have to necessarily believe what you explore, just suspend your disbelief for a while. You will be amazed what untapped potential awaits when you:

- Explore homeopathy;
- Explore clinical nutrition;
- Explore chiropractic treatment;
- Explore osteopathic medicine;
- Explore botanical medicine;
- Explore ayurvedic teachings and principles;
- Explore Rife frequencies and the principles of resonance;
- Explore pulsed electromagnetic field therapies, such as Medithera;
- Explore meditation and the science of heart coherence;
- Explore energy healing methods, such as:
    Reconnective Healing with Dr. Eric Pearl,
    Matrix Energetics with Dr. Richard Bartlett,
    Emotional Freedom Technques with Gary Craig
    Tapas Acupressure Technique with Tapas Fleming
    Pan-Gu Shengong with Master Ou;
- If you suffer with drug addiction, you might want to explore treatment with Iboga or ibogaine. Iboga is a plant medicine from Gabon, Africa and used by the Bwiti tribes. Ibogaine is a semi-synthetic single alkaloid derivative of the whole root extract. Both have extremely high rates of success in treating addiction to street drugs, such as heroin and crack, as well as prescription drugs and SSRIs; or
- Perhaps you are drawn to healing through another cultural model, such as a curandero or shaman of South America. There are those who have experienced physical and emotional

healing through the use of ayahuasca, San Pedro and other similar plant medicines. Just because they may be outside of your cultural familiarity does not mean they do not work.

Having explored *all* of the methods mentioned above, I have seen many miraculous healings and recoveries in conditions that were deemed "hopeless" by conventional medical perspectives, including everything from heavy heroin addiction to healing from PTSD and depression!

There are a number of excellent books, authors and videos that can help explain some of the general concepts and quantum physics principles underlying energy healing. Dr. Edgar Mitchell, who walked on the moon during the Apollo 14 mission, founded the Institute of Noetic Sciences and has openly shared his personal experiences with energy healing and consciousness research. Our emerging understanding of quantum physics, including principles of bi-location, quantum entanglement, the observer effect and others, have provided a perspective of how things are, beyond the old Newtonian physics. I have provided a number of resources in Appendix B for your consideration and on the web site. Whether you choose to apply any energy healing methodologies or not, you will benefit from your wider understanding of yourself and your place in this universe. Such an understanding is empowering and effectively counteracts the victimization attitude inherent in modern medicine.

The first two suggestions that follow are arguably the most important and the most powerful steps one can take toward greater Consciousness, greater personal power and improved health. They are, in fact, two sides of the same coin and have to do with reclaiming control over your inner space and eliminating the external programming. Each issue outlined below has the potential to enhance or improve your health, both directly and indirectly. Some issues will be more important for some readers than others, depending on your state of awareness and your current perspective. I would encourage you to pause for a moment after reading each topic to reflect on how your life might be improved by adopting such a change in perspective or habit.

Meditation and Heart Coherence: One of the most powerful things you can do not only for yourself but also for the people around you is to adopt a daily practice that strengthens your internal self-management skills. Doing so might be through daily meditation or heart coherence. Either practice will help quiet the mind and allow space for the voice of Consciousness to be heard. It adds resilience to our physiology, reduces over-reactivity and behaves as the antidote to daily stresses. Research shows that heart coherence improves creativity and problem-solving ability, enhances intuition and supports a sense of inner peace. When you are in alignment and in a healthy energy flow, your state of well-being affects the people around you. This impact has been studied for over twenty years and has been shown to be a powerful, multifaceted practice capable of improving many aspects of our lives and health. The links provided in the Resource section on the MindMythsBook.com website can guide you to the research literature and applications.

"Who looks outside, dreams. Who looks inside, awakens." – Carl Jung

Television and MSM: If you live in the United States, you have already realized that most of what we refer to as "Main Stream Media" (MSM) is little more than distracting, largely irrelevant entertainment. The System uses this programming to keep you in their box, focused on their agenda, not yours. If you were to visualize National Public Radio (NPR) as one goal post on the playing field and, say, Fox News as the other goal post, the name of the game is to keep you within the goal posts. By implication, going out of bounds from their defined playing field may cause you to be subjected to ridicule and derision from friends, family and neighbors who are still playing the System's game. In some countries, there is no pretext of choice in media; there is one channel, and the government decides what gets aired and what is censored. Unplugging from television and the conventional media is a powerful and far-reaching step toward deprogramming your mind and your beliefs. While keeping informed about world events is important to many people, it can be easily argued that MSM does not even do that honestly or accurately. You can easily obtain your fix of news and world information from numerous independent sources, many of which you access via the Internet. Addiction to television as a constant noise in the background might be a challenge to eliminate, but doing so is well worth the effort.

The Anger Trap: As I mentioned in the Introduction, people are awakening, and many are doing so into a state of anger. Anger feels like a perfectly appropriate and justified response when we realize the level of deception and control under which we have lived. Anger is frequently the response we create when we feel our boundaries have been violated and we wish to reassert them. Yet anger will not help find a solution unless we can successfully channel that energy into positive action, lest we fall unwittingly into the Hegelian trap of problem, reaction and solution. (Refer back to Chapter 6 if you need a refresher on Hegelian dialectics.) John Lennon wisely cautioned against anger and violence against the System when he said, "When it gets down to having to use violence, then you are playing the system's game. The establishment will irritate you—pull your beard, flick your face—to make you fight. Because once they've got you violent, then they know how to handle you. The only thing they don't know how to handle is non-violence and humor."

Vote Strategically: Yes, your vote surely does count, but I am not talking about your vote at the ballot box for an elected office. I am speaking here of your commercial vote. From first-world countries to third-world countries, we all live in a world that has become dominated and subsumed by commerce. Commerce has become part of almost everything we do, from going to a movie and to purchasing food to taking a taxi and receiving some compensation for the work you perform. Whether you use the dollar, peso, euro, rupee, pound or other currency, you possess the power to shape and mold the world around you. If you wish to see more organic foods in your local stores, then vote for more organic foods by purchasing them. If you wish to see more alternative health practitioners in your area, vote for more by making them successful and supporting their practices. If you wish to see your local community thrive and local mom-and-pop shops become successful, then vote for them by shopping there rather than frequenting the big-box stores that suck the profits out to off-shore destinations. If you value the personal attention of your locally owned pharmacy, hardware store or market, vote for them with your dollars. The only reason that natural medicine has gained some acceptance (or at least tolerance) by the conventional medical system and made significant inroads into the popular consciousness is because people wanted it and voted for more of it with their purchases. Stores and supermarkets will sell whatever sells as long as they can make a profit. Selling food is a business! Whether they sell sugary cupcakes or organic carrots really matters not to them. It matters to *you*. It matters to all of us. Vote wisely. Vote for your future, not merely for price, because the money you think you save will cost you more dearly in the future. And if you believe that your vote at the ballot box does matter and does represent choice, then by all means, vote there as well. Having power is meaningless unless you are willing to use it wisely.

Whatever social or commercial system people find themselves in and whether they believe that to be a fair or just system, is largely a product of what they have allowed to be. The notable orator, statesman and former slave Frederick Douglas once stated: "Find out just what any people will quietly submit to and you have the exact measure of the injustice and wrong which will be imposed on them". Through conscious choice and right action, positive change can be manifest. It is a choice.

The "Rescue Me" Syndrome: The number of adults who remain passive and inactive in their health care, even when their condition is serious, is surprising. While there can be a number of reasons for being disengaged, one common reason may be an unspoken desire to be rescued from their illness. I have seen many sick and suffering people waste precious time waiting until the so-called experts develop the vaccine for their virus, or develop the next supposed wonder drug to treat their fibromyalgia or diabetes. What they really want is to be rescued. Colette Dowling coined the term "Cinderella complex" and wrote a bestselling book in 1990 by the same name; in it, she discusses a fear of independence in women and an unconscious desire to be taken care of by others. In this case, the theme of the Cinderella complex can be aptly applied to matters of health for both genders. Yielding to this unconscious desire to be cured without personal effort or involvement can be devastating and result in years of continued illness and suffering. Healing is always a journey—*your* journey. You only have to look at the US and the dismal results from the public policy supported "War on Cancer", initiated way back in 1971, to see what happens when we wait for someone else to find the answers.

Be Skeptical, But Learn to Listen: This is actually the Fifth Agreement from the book by the same title, written by Don Miguel Ruiz. This immensely valuable perspective can be a major help in breaking our conditioned response to reject that which we have been told is not possible. Doing so allows us to explore new ideas and options that come our way and, through personal research and investigation, see what is true. The Toltec were an indigenous Mesoamerican culture centered mainly in central Mexico and in the Toltec teachings, beliefs are seen as a kind of foggy lens through which we view our world, and they affect our ability to see the truth without bias or distortion. When searching for answers in our personal health, whether for something we interpret as a physical problem or an emotional problem, we do best when we can see all of our options and opportunities. "Be Skeptical but Learn to Listen" is the axiom born of vision and wisdom that frees us from our own limiting beliefs and those imposed by others. Don Miguel Ruiz was born in Mexico. Intrigued by Western science and medicine, he trained as a surgeon after attending medical school. But after a near-death experience shook his life, he undertook a long process of introspection and self-discovery. Born into a family of healers, he returned to his ancestral home to study with his mother, a curandera (healer), and his grandfather, a nagual (shaman). Based on his personal crisis and journey of discovery, he brings forward this ancient knowledge. In an effort to help free others from limiting beliefs, Don Miguel is inclined to say, "Don't believe me, don't believe anyone else, don't believe yourself."

The Magic of a New "What If…?": It is clear that altering our perspective can be one of the most powerful changes we can make. In some cases, simply asking ourselves a carefully worded question or two can start the process whenever you are ready. Question number one is, "What if I already have everything I need to be happy at this very moment?" When we ask ourselves this question, we bring to consciousness the idea that our state of happiness may not be related to a supposed lack of some external circumstance or thing and that, in fact, we can be happy right now if we choose to see it that way. If we have unconsciously adopted the belief of "I'll be happy when…" (such as when I have children, when I have the right job, when I find the right relationship or fill in the blank!), we will never find happiness, because the mind will always find something else it wants and another reason to remain unfulfilled. Many ancient teachings state that we create our happiness moment by moment. Such a belief is the essence of self-empowerment.

The other "What if…" question we can ask is: "What if I already have everything I need to be healthy at this moment?" This question parallels the one above, of course, and helps open our thought processes to look anew at what we already know and can already do for ourselves. You do not have to believe that the premise of the question is true:

just ask the question anyway. This may aptly apply to the diabetic who *knows* that eating a bowl of ice cream before bed is not a healthy choice but chooses to do so anyway. Or, to the fibromyalgia patient who stays up past midnight each night to get a few more things done *knowing* that pre-midnight sleep is critical to self-repair and recovery. Or to the migraine sufferer, who understands their personal cause-and-effect relationship between eating cheese and drinking wine and the onset of a migraine the next day but chooses to indulge anyway. In each case, they already possess that which they need to be healthy, but *choose* not to see it.

An important feature of asking either of these two powerful questions is that you do not have to believe that either one is true. No, you do not have to believe that you already have everything you need to be happy for the question to have its effect. The act of asking the question and being open to a new answer creates its own effects. If you practice asking these questions, you may eventually choose to see them as truth. But as an exercise in perspective shifting, they can truly change your world!

Dare to Express Your Uniqueness and Let Others Do the Same: In every society or group, the internal drive for uniqueness confronts society's pressure to conform. Even in societies that profess a belief in diversity and individuality, conformity is usually the goal. But how can you evolve to become the truly magnificent *you* that you are if you are expected to adopt the attitudes, beliefs and roles created by others? How can you allow yourself to be unique if you are uncomfortable with the uniqueness of others? How many people speak about the wonders of diversity but only to the extent that it is practiced within the confines of their accepted norms and values? The famous British philosopher Alan Watts once said that "insecure societies are the most intolerant of 'non-joiners'… they are so unsure of the validity of their game rules that they say everyone must play." As you reclaim your personal power and discover who you really are, you will necessarily change. These changes in you may make others around you a bit uncomfortable, especially if they have known you for a while. The reverse is true as well: in allowing yourself to grow and change, extend that same allowance to others.

Gossip: Gossip is the most basic of human languages and is perhaps the most universally spoken. However, it is also the cruelest, the most judgmental and the most unjust form of communication. It is based on rumors, half-truths and hearsay, and the party about which you speak is not even present to correct the misperceptions. By making the conscious choice to disengage from gossip, we move toward restoring honesty and integrity in our word. When we opt out of gossip, we may have fewer words to speak, but those words can now take on greater meaning. By our choice of language and word-symbols, we can support a culture of justice, fairness, privacy and kindness. If you recall the earlier discussion about how sound affects form in cymatics (refer back to Chapter 10 for a refresher on cymatics) you will appreciate that your words affect you and others.

Drama: Many people live for and through the drama in their lives: drama in their relationships, at work, within the family and everywhere else. Yes, stuff happens in life, but for some people the drama has *become* life, not something in the way of living life. Drama is like the static on the radio or the short circuit in the computer. It is noise without information, volume without meaning and attention without purpose. Drama is also stress without purpose. Some people unconsciously create an endless stream of drama to avoid facing the bigger issues in life and the discomfort that results from being quiet and alone with themselves and their thoughts. Drama can be a device that allows people to focus on others and avoid facing themselves. Examine your day-to-day living and see if you are using drama or creating drama as a substitute for substance and meaning. How much less stress could you be experiencing each day and each week if you disengaged from the drama? If you recall our discussion about how stress keeps us in a state of "fight or flight" and chronic disrepair, you can once again appreciate how drama works against our physical and mental health. Leonardo da Vinci once stated that "Where there is shouting, there is no true knowledge" and that seems no less true today.

Control: Letting go of the need to be in control can be quite liberating. The idea that we can actually be in control of the events of life is an illusion that only generates frustration and discord. More than likely, you would not welcome an effort by someone else to control you, so why would you want to control them? Rather than exerting great emotional and mental energy attempting to control people or events around you, work to adjust your perceptions of people and events and thus your reactions to both. This suggestion is not to say that you have to *like* everything that comes your way in life, you just don't have to control it. I like the perspective offered by Byron Katie in *Loving What Is* when she said, "I can find only three kinds of business in the universe: mine, yours and God's. Much of our stress comes from mentally living out of our business." By liberating yourself from a need to be in control, you can greatly lessen the level of frustration and internal discord you experience when people and events don't go as you desired.

Blaming: Things happen and not always in accordance your immediate desires and personal plans. Rather than blaming others for what happens to you or for what you have or do not have, or for what you are feeling or not feeling, look to your *self* to see what you can learn from the experience or how you can change your perspective. Very often we learn *more* from what we think of as our failures than from our successes. Should a smoker blame the cigarettes or his physician or the tobacco companies when there was a choice to smoke? When we blame, we are giving our power to other people or events. When we blame, we are less likely to learn from the experience, and are thus more likely to experience it again. Accepting our part in the way of things not only allows us to grow but also liberates us from seeing ourselves as a helpless victim.

Quiet the Mind Chatter: As we said earlier, you have roughly 60,000 thoughts in a day, and 80% are negative or reinforce a negative belief. With time, awareness and gentle patience, you can quiet that negative chatter and disallow it to run away with your mind. Understanding that the chatter voice in your head is *not* really you can also help. Negative mind-chatter is the product of old programming from the early years of your life that probably does not serve you now. Why carry it? You may find the techniques known as Emotional Freedom Techniques (EFT) and / or the Tapas Acupressure Technique (TAT) very helpful to erase the really entrenched negative programs, but awareness is the first step. It is also a matter of practicing and learning how to quiet the mind. How much of our daily distress arises from that incessant stream of chatter in our heads? In many traditions, finding peace in the mind is the gateway to finding peace in the body and in life.

Complaining and Criticizing: You know who they are, and they are no joy to be around. But for some people, complaining and criticizing is a way of life. It is as if they see the glass as always half-empty Criticizing and complaining does nothing to improve your situation or provide solutions to problems; it just strengthens the pattern of seeing the negative in all things. If all you see and talk about is what you *don't* like, then you will only see more of what you don't like. Here is a good rule of thumb: Offer your opinion, assistance or advice *only* if you are requested to do so and then give it, honestly and with integrity. Everyone knows you have an opinion, so if you are not asked to share it, then consider remaining silent.

Dump the Guilt: Carrying guilt can be as heavy a burden as carrying a backpack filled with eighty pounds of gravel. Guilt zaps our energy and stifles new learning. Guilt is all about the past. Instead of feeling guilty, we can learn to accept responsibility for whatever we feel guilty about, realize that as an adult we will make mistakes and errors in judgment as part of our journey and then let it *go*. Often we learn more from our mistakes and failures than our successes; in all actuality, if we learn from these events, have we really failed? Know inside that you absolutely did the best you could have done with what you knew at the time and under the circumstance you found yourself. Had you known differently at the time or had a crystal ball into the future, you might have chosen differently. But maybe not. No one can see all possible outcomes, and no one is so wise that they do not make mistakes. As mentioned above, if you are feeling "stuck", then seek the help of a professional and explore EFT and TAT as methods of releasing what no longer serves you.

Seeing the World Through Labels: As we discussed previously, labels are merely symbols that we use in a crude attempt to categorize people, things and even other symbols. When we invest our energy in symbols, we lose our own power. While the use of labels often appears to be a practical way to categorize things and people in our world, such symbols are frequently misleading and are often charged with subliminal content that can distort reality. Symbols can be used to unite or divide, to inform or confuse, to inspire or intimidate. Categorizing people according to their skin color, spiritual beliefs, political ideology or ethnicity keeps us all divided along meaningless and frequently manufactured lines of division. This tendency toward labeling is analogous to two astronauts standing on the moon arguing over which spacesuit is superior, the silver one or the white one. Do we really want to define the substance of a man or woman by the color of the spacesuit they live in or by the un-chosen geography of their birth? Is this not the essence of the divide-and-rule policy and the antithesis of peaceful cooperation? If you look carefully, you will see how frequently and gently the System and the media in particular encourage people to divide themselves into factions. Whether the division is caused by class warfare epitomized by "tax the rich to help the poor", a cultural/ethnic division of "Latino" versus "Caucasian", a racial division of "black versus white" or even through the innocence of regional sports teams strengthening the clan mentality of "us versus them", divisions keep people squabbling and distracted rather then uniting and building.

The most effective tool to create division among people is fear. Just look how frequently in history governments have created an enemy, a boogeyman if you will, to instill fear in the population to justify new controls. Fear can also arise from natural or manmade disasters, including hurricanes, economic crises and so on. But we also know that the antithesis of "divide and rule" is "love and community", the Achilles' heel of any system of centralized control. Love is the antidote to the constant messages of fear: fear of lurking terrorists, distrust or suspicion of your neighbor, the constant worry about your family's safety or general fear about the future. Community, then, is the antidote to division. Getting to know your neighbors, shopping at locally owned shops, utilizing local services, supporting charity efforts that serve your neighbors and treating the people you meet with a smile, a look in the eye and heartfelt "hello" are expressions and actions we can all take *immediately* that strengthen the fabric of community and, ultimately, our lives.

Think for a moment what an incredibly dynamic and healthy world we could create if we got past the labels! What progress, peace and freedom might we experience if we could learn to see people for who and what they are individually, and not as a group?

Eliminating Excuses: More often than not, we make excuses to try to make ourselves feel better or to justify our behaviors. Excuses are really lies we tell ourselves and others, and a lie only has power when someone believes it. The truth is just the truth, whether anyone believes it or not. Truth can stand for itself. If you are stuck in a pattern of behavior or speech that requires repeated excuses, pause and take a look at what is really going on. As someone once said, "A lie may take care of the present, but it has no future." Being truthful with yourself is one of the greatest gifts you can give to yourself, to those around you and to your community, and it is a source of tremendous personal power. Learn to use it.

Releasing Resentments: It has been said that resentment is like drinking poison and waiting for the other person to die. Holding onto old grudges only corrodes you and your soul. The party you are angry with is probably not losing sleep over *your* issue. So forgiveness is something you do for *yourself*, not for them. Forgiving releases you from your burden, pain and suffering. It is not just a "head thing" that you say to yourself; it is the release of all the stored energy and emotion that goes with the particular event. The act of forgiveness can seem to be an insurmountable challenge in some circumstances. But sometimes the scars and wounds go too deep and for those who feel stuck and need help, Emotional Freedom Technique (EFT) can be a life-changer when we are totally imprisoned by certain emotional patterns. There are DVD materials available, and certified EFT practitioners can guide you in this remarkable healing technique.

Letting Go of Attachments: In many affluent societies, acquiring "stuff" seems to be a big part of life. At least, that is how it first appears. We are influenced and programmed by television, media and the people in our lives that we need to get "stuff." Who wouldn't want an expansive wardrobe and sharp clothes, a couple of nice new cars in the garage, the latest smartphone, iThis or iThat and so on? We tend to define our lives and our successes by the stuff we accumulate, and we can feel powerful by the fact that we *can* accumulate it. But you are you with or without your stuff, and there is an inherent danger in allowing the material goods we enjoy to obscure our true identity. Try this little experiment and ask yourself this question: "What could I take from my life and still be me?" Think about all the stuff you have. Select one item and take it away. After you answer that question once, ask the question again. And again. What can you take out of your life and still be you? If you do this honestly, it can be quite revealing and liberating. One of the surprise lessons that people with a lot of stuff frequently come to learn is that the stuff actually owns *you*. You have to take care of it, winterize it, insure it, clean it, wax it, fix it, polish it, remodel it, heat it, cool it, store it, etc. All of that takes great energy and additional resources of time and money.

But stuff is not the only object of attachment. We can become attached to our appearance, our hairstyle, being viewed by others as an expert or anything that we habitually feel we need to bolster a sense of feeling good about ourselves. As you walk through your day, start to take note of things that you have really become attached to. What do these things mean to you? Why? What would happen if you were suddenly without them? How much of your power have you put into these attachments, and are they serving your higher purpose? You will come to see what you need to do.

Ghosts of the Past: We all have a history, and everyone has their story. We all move through life experience by experience. Some experiences are positive and pleasant, while some are traumatic and terrible. We do not always have a voice in choosing the events, but we do have choice in how we react. Nevertheless, those events and experiences have contributed to who we are, how we think and how we interact with our world. How we respond to those experiences may be positive or negative, healthy or unhealthy. I have listened to people still defining their experience today by the ex-husband they divorced twenty years earlier. Or perhaps they still recite the story of the girlfriend that dumped them over ten years ago? Or the 55-year-old man who loves to talk about his high school days when he was the hero on the football team. We cannot grow into what we can become when we drag that huge sack of past experiences around with us. Placing our power in experiences of the past denies us our power today. Reclaim it.

Building a Library of Self-Help Skills: A large contributor to feeling empowered is having both a perspective and set of skills that can support us through the changes and challenges of life. Finding peace and a sense of fulfillment in life is about first finding these qualities inside ourselves. When you have adopted a daily practice meditation or heart coherence, when you can skillfully work with EFT for the benefit of yourself or others, when you have a healthy sense of "your business, their business and God's business", then you have acquired an ability to support your growth and the expansion of your own Consciousness. One of my favorite quotations is from Gandhi: "Be the change you wish to see in the world"! If we wish to see justice in the world, then we can start by treating our own bodies with justice. If we wish to see peace in the world, we must first create that peace within. If we wish for greater freedom in our lives, we can free ourselves from the limiting beliefs we hold and from the attempt to control our life and the lives of others.

Each of the concepts outlined above represents a powerful potential for change, and the key to transcending chronic illness is by transforming our selves. By examining and implementing each of the steps outlined above, you can effect powerful changes in your physiology. Whether you are lowering your stress levels and allowing your body to move into "rest and repair" mode or liberating yourself from anger, resentment or the distracting drama of life, you are creating a new environment for each of the 50 trillion cells that comprise your physical body. By changing how you react to people and events, you are changing your neurochemistry. By understanding the neurology axiom of "neurons that fire together, wire together" you can create new, healthier patterns of being. As you reflect on each of the suggestions outlined above, note whether you feel any special *affinity for* or *resistance to* any particular step. If so, you may want to devote extra thought and research into that issue and explore what it means for you.

Physician and writer Deepak Chopra speaks of the power of past conditioning in these important words: "In detachment lies the wisdom of uncertainty... in the wisdom of uncertainty lies the freedom from our past, from the known, which is the prison of past conditioning. And in our willingness to step into the unknown, the field of all possibilities, we surrender ourselves to the creative mind that orchestrates the dance of the universe".

By shedding the beliefs originating from lack, limitation and helplessness, you can reacquire the power you were meant to have. By seeing past the illusions presented to you, you can create a new reality. In the process, you may discover that the most powerful forces in your life are **fear**, **belief** and **love**.

Chapter 37

Daily Action Steps

"Truth resides in every human heart, and one has to search for it there, and to be guided by truth as one sees it. But no one has a right to coerce others to act according to his own view of truth." – Mahatma Gandhi

Fortunately there are many levels upon which we can act to alter the flow of power back to our Self. Simply remember that much of what we do to regain our power and our freedom is apophatic in nature, through our use of the Word of Power: *no*.

1. Start each day by focusing your energy and your consciousness with twenty minutes of quiet meditation, contemplation, prayer, heart coherence or whatever technique you prefer to create internal balance and harmony. Make this action as regular as brushing your teeth or combing your hair;
2. Join a CSA (community-supported agriculture) and/or a co-op to purchase much of your food;
3. Support local farming and local farm stands, especially organic farming enterprises;
4. Pay for your food items with your local paper and coin currency as much as possible, rather than electronic credit;
5. Stop using a supermarket savings card. The so-called discount you receive is actually your payment for their right to sell your purchasing information to anyone they choose;

6. Take prescriptions, when they are necessary, to a small, independent pharmacy rather than the large national chain pharmacies who sell your information out the back door;
7. Make it your personal policy to get copies of *all* medical tests, reports, scans, etc. after each visit with your physician. You should be the keeper of your health information, which is especially critical of you ever have a medical error that holds the potential for litigation or, in greater likelihood, you simply want a true second opinion;
8. Find a physician who respects your beliefs regarding vaccinations and is open to working with you in an adult-to-adult manner;
9. If you are considering any vaccine, be sure to do your *own* research! There are numerous independent books and web sites that can provide the critical information you need to make a responsible decision. Read the vaccine package insert, which you can get online or from a pharmacy. Find out about the preservatives and the adjuvants, as well as whether the vaccine contains mercury, aluminum or phenol. See the Resources appendix for additional information;
10. If you live in the United States, you can write to the MIB Group, Inc. and request a copy of the medical information file they have created on you. MIB Group is a private data collection company owned by 470 or so insurance companies that collects and shares information about you. Do you know what they are saying? Do you know what information they are sharing? See www.mib.com for more information;
11. If you want to make a difference in future medical care, support those practitioners who are already providing superior care or the type of care you wish to see more of. If

you wish to support the funding of alternative research, find a group that defends the freedom of those already doing that research. Before you join the next so-called walk for the cure or sport the latest colored ribbon, check out where donated money actually goes. How much money actually goes to research or patient care? What percentage of the money collected is used for overhead expenses, salaries, trips and such? Is this just a front to collect more money for BigPharma? You may not be supporting what you really believe in;

12. If you have an upcoming important medical appointment, bring someone who can "speak medical" if you are not knowledgeable in medicine or biology. This person might be a friend who is a nurse, physician's assistant or someone who has a grasp of medicine and how to phrase important questions. If possible, prepare your questions in advance so you know what you want to get from your visit. If you need more time to get all your questions answered, ask to schedule additional time with the physician when such a discussion is possible;

13. Always get a second or third opinion when major health or medical decisions are pending. When obtaining a true second opinion, avoid biasing your second opinion practitioner with the information from the first opinion provider. You want an *unbiased* second opinion, not a rubber stamp. If possible, get that second or third opinion from a medical provider in another state or region where it is highly unlikely that he or she knows, has lunch with or plays golf with your first-opinion physician;

14. If you have experienced trauma in life and it continues to affect your current well-being, find a practitioner who is well-trained in Emotional Freedom Technique (EFT), Tapas Acupressure Technique (TAT) or another effective tapping

method to help neutralize the neural and energetic imprint that trauma leaves behind. When used skillfully, these techniques can be highly effective with post-traumatic stress disorder (PTSD) and have helped many veterans who have suffered for years;

15. Acquire some good natural medicine home first-aid books and familiarize yourself with them. This material may include first-aid books on homeopathy, herbal medicine, etc. A few consultations with a clinical nutritionist or naturopath can also help educate you in first-aid and self-care for acute illnesses. The intent is not to replace appropriate medical care when needed, but to empower you to deal with the smaller issues and prevent them from becoming larger medical issues;

16. Take steps to assure that the air and water in your home environment are clean and free of fluoride and other chemicals;

17. Become aware of devices that create electromagnetic fields (EMF) in your home and take steps to keep them at a healthy distance from locations where you may sit or sleep. These devices may include power boxes to a home or apartment, televisions, cordless phones and so on. If necessary, invest in a reasonably good EMF meter to make the invisible visible and know where high-field readings occur within your home;

18. Avoid all non-critical x-ray and high-intensity radiation exposure. This exposure would include non-critical medical x-rays, CT scans, ultrasounds and MRIs. Make all such decisions on a carefully considered case-by-case basis;

19. Opt out of the full-body scanners at airports, bus stations, train stations or wherever they are being used. Independent studies show that neither the tetrahertz (millimeter wave) technology nor the x-ray radiation are safe (tetrahertz

radiation shreds DNA). Independent experts have voiced concerns that, because these devices are not being used within a medical setting, there is little if any monitoring or calibration, and the amount of radiation received may be more than is safe.

Chapter 38

Personal Action Steps

Privacy is a key personal power. Privacy is not about secrecy, but about having the power and the freedom to control those aspects of your life related to who you are, where you go and what you do. Unfortunately, privacy appears to be a vanishing right, frequently because people do not understand it or value it.

This trend toward lack of privacy is contrary to the natural progression observed by Ayn Rand, who said, "Civilization is the progress toward a society of privacy. The savage's whole existence is public, ruled by the laws of his tribe. Civilization is the process of setting man free from men."

Privacy is the primary obstacle to centralized control, manipulation and ultimately abuse. Valuing privacy does not suggest a desire to hide or engage in clandestine activities. It merely means you value your privacy. Having nothing to hide is not the point. It is more about who controls the informational aspects of your life and not inviting abuse. Many believe privacy is an inherent right of all peoples. What do you believe?

Here are some things that you can do to protect your privacy:

- Use your domestic paper and coin currency for purchases whenever possible, rather than electronic means such as credit cards. The advantage is privacy, and by using cash you are not enriching the banks through the merchant fees they collect from the seller. Using cash is the antithesis of centralization; it de funds the System, and banks cannot hypothecate more debt against it;

- Consider eliminating the use of that automated toll taker from your car windshield. Many countries now have them in busy metropolitan areas. It not only makes it too convenient to collect the toll, but the transponders can locate your position all along highways, and not just at tollbooths. Such location data is commonly subpoenaed in legal proceedings to prove where people were and when;

- Use a proxy, VPN or other privacy feature or software to maintain your online privacy;

- Use an email provider service that respects privacy. As of this writing, Gmail, Google, some cloud services and many other providers of supposedly free email services say they actively profile and share information about you and your communications. Read their privacy policy very carefully before signing up. For many, there is no privacy offered, and, in fact, you do not know where your personal information is going or how it is being used;

- Keep your driver's license and all credit or debit cards that are embedded with smart chips in a metal sleeve or pouch to prevent thieves with scanners from reading your private data contained on the RFID chip. The same concern would apply to many new passports that contain an RFID chip;

- Use a private mailbox or post office box for all mail, and use that address on checks, accounts and so on. Doing so helps keep your home a place of privacy and refuge from the commercial world;

- Be discreet and learn to watch what you say in emails and other Internet communications. They are not private or secure means of communication. Highly charged emotional statements or threats you really do not mean could get you in trouble;

- If you need to transmit sensitive personal, medical or business information via email, then use one of many encryption programs that allow for safe, encrypted communications. Assume that anything you say in an unsecure email is open to the world;

- Get out of or greatly reduce your presence in any social networking sites you have joined. If you must be involved, be *very careful* about what you say about yourself and be cautious about inadvertently violating the privacy of others. Some people may strongly object to having their name mentioned, having their personal information disclosed, appearing in photos or being spoken about in social messages. Social web sites are data mining operations for various intelligence agencies, law enforcement and criminals, and what goes into these systems can never be erased, even if you close your account. The more information you release from your control, the greater the opportunity for the unscrupulous to misuse it;

- Get an anonymous or junk email address for subscriptions or blind inquiries and use this email address when you do not know exactly who you are dealing with. There are many such providers. You do not need to be profiled;

- Find three or four good alternative news sources online to get an independent, non-system perspective on national and global events. (Some suggestions are provided in the

Resources appendix.) No matter what country you live in, news reports from other countries about what is happening in your nation can provide very different information than what you might receive from your domestic television or print sources. Learn to read between the lines and question what you see and hear; and

- Better yet, turn off the television news and *stop* the programming. Television programming is the essence of what the System needs and wants you to believe. Protect your mind, thoughts and sanity. It is time to deprogram yourself!

The power contained within the suggestions outlined above cannot be overemphasized. When we change ourselves, we change our health, our life and our world. It is a concept embodied in these words by Mahatma Gandhi: "If we could change ourselves, the tendencies in the world would also change. As a man changes his own nature, so does the attitude of the world change towards him. ... We need not wait to see what others do."

In Appendix B, I have listed a number of resources from which you can start or expand your journey and your understanding. The list is not exhaustive, but rather one by which you can easily start moving forward.

Part VII

Epilogue

> Your beliefs become your thoughts,
> Your thoughts become your words,
> Your words become your actions,
> Your actions become your habits,
> Your habits become your values,
> Your values become your destiny.
> Mahatma Gandhi

Our journey together during the course of this discussion has taken us into the world of myths, perceptions, power and identity. We have examined how we think and process new information as well as some of the important concepts and forces that we each experience through the course of our daily lives. Ultimately, we all seek health, vitality, resilience, abundance, a sense of purpose, a desire to be appreciated and loved, to experience a sense of belonging and to possess that special, sometimes elusive quality of inner peace. Why we and so many of our brothers and sisters living around the world as fellow, creative Conscious beings do not experience these attributes has been the focus of our discussion. We come to realize that when we change our perspective, we change what we value and how we value it. As Albert Einstein once said: "Not everything that counts can be counted, and not everything that can be counted counts".

Perhaps these pages have helped you to understand who you really are and the magnificent potential that you inherently possess. Perhaps you have come to the conclusion that as the masterful creator of your life, the real you is Consciousness itself and that Consciousness is timeless. Perhaps you also realize that up until now, you have not fully appreciated your own power and that you were enticed to lend or surrender it to others. Perhaps if each of us is willing to abandon the perspective of lack, limitation and scarcity, then we can join together in creating a better world; a world based on health, beauty, peace, freedom and abundance. Perhaps we can see past the symbols and the artificial labels that keep us divided and mired in conflict. Perhaps now you realize that reclaiming your power can transform your health, your life and ultimately the world. As you may now realize, this is ultimately a revolution in Consciousness and an evolution in Consciousness occurring at the same time, and you are invited to become part of it by making the choice to do so.

It is my sincere hope that something within these pages has served as a catalyst to inspire, motivate and accelerate you along your path to total wellness. To do so would be my greatest joy.

There is a wonderful quote from *A Return to Love: Reflections on the Principles of A Course in Miracles* by Marianne Williamson that I wish to leave you with that really speaks to the essence of the message within these pages.

> Our deepest fear is not that we are inadequate. Our deepest fear is that we are powerful beyond measure. It is our light, not our darkness that most frightens us. ….And as we let

our own light shine, we unconsciously give other people permission to do the same. As we are liberated from our own fear, our presence automatically liberates others.

~ The Beginning ~

Peace and Blessings,

Jeffery Scott

Glossary

Allopathic/allopathy: relating to a philosophy and system of medicine where interventions are designed to combat disease by using drugs or surgery intended to produce the opposite of what the body is experiencing. Origin: 1842, "treatment of disease by remedies that produce effects opposite to the symptoms," from the German *Allopathie* a term coined by Samuel Hahnemann the father of modern homeopathy) Example: taking a drug to help move your bowels when constipated or a drug to slow your bowels when you have diarrhea.

Chiropractic: a system of therapeutics based primarily upon the importance of the interaction of the spine, the nervous system and associated organs. Treatment is designed to manually adjust or align the segments of the spinal column.

Clinical Nutrition: The discipline of human clinical nutrition applies principles derived from current biochemical and physiological scientific knowledge for the purpose of promoting optimal health while recognizing biochemical individuality. Therapeutic protocols may include: nutrition/lifestyle modification, nutritive supplementation, detoxification support, understanding of physiological/biochemical pathways and support for the body's innate regenerative processes.

Cognitive Dissonance: the anxiety and discomfort that results from attempting to simultaneously hold contradictory or otherwise incompatible attitudes, beliefs or experiences, such as when one likes a person but disapproves strongly of one of his or her habits.

Hegelian Dialectics: a framework for guiding thoughts and actions to a predetermined solution through the use of a created or exploited problem (the thesis) and a coordinated vocal opposition to the problem (the reaction/antithesis) leading to the resulting and desired solution (the synthesis). For example, Mary states that 3 + 2 = 7 (a problem). Sam asserts (reaction) that 3 + 2 = 5. The synthesis (solution) between the two opposing points of view is to agree that 3 + 2 = 6. Hegelian dialectics is premised on the idea that the truth lies somewhere in the middle.

Homeopathic/homeopathy: relating to a philosophy and method of treating disease by the use of exceedingly small amounts of a substance that, in healthy persons, produces symptoms similar to those of the disease being treated. The "remedies", as they are called, are prepared by a special process called "succussion", which is a process of serial dilution and vigorous shaking of the preparation.

Learned Helplessness: the act of giving up trying as a result of either consistent failure to be rewarded in life or a sense of inability to escape an adverse situation. Thought to be a cause of depression.

Naturopathic/naturopathy: relating to a philosophy and system of treating illness without the use of surgery or synthetic drugs but utilizing special diets, herbs, remedies, vitamins, massage, etc. to assist the body's natural healing processes.

Osteopathy: a system and philosophy of health care that separated from the allopathic medical model more than a century ago. Osteopathy places emphasis on the musculoskeletal system and is based on a presumption that an energy flow exists between the musculoskeletal system and the organs and that such a flow is vital to health. Osteopaths believe strongly in the innate healing power of the body and do their best to facilitate that strength. The discipline originated in 1890s with the work of Dr. Andrew Taylor and has similarities with chiropractic.

Stockholm Syndrome: a psychological and emotional attachment to a captor formed by one held hostage typically as a result of continuous stress, dependence and/or a need to cooperate for survival.

Appendix A

Excerpts from United States Senate document number 264, 1936:

> The alarming fact is that foods-fruits and vegetables-grains now being raised on millions of acres of land that no longer contains enough of certain minerals, are starving us...no matter how much of them we eat!

> This talk of minerals is novel and quite startling. In fact, a realization of the importance of minerals in food is so new that the textbooks on nutritional dietetics contain very little about it. Nevertheless it is something that concerns all of us, and the further we delve into it the more startling it becomes.

> Laboratory tests prove that the fruits, the vegetables, the grains, the eggs and even the milk and meats of today are not what they were a few generations ago. No man of today can eat enough fruits and vegetables to supply his system with the minerals he requires for perfect health...

> No longer does a balanced and fully nourishing diet consist merely of so many calories or certain vitamins or a fixed proportion of starches, proteins, and carbohydrates. We now know that it must contain, in addition, something like a score of trace minerals.

It is bad news to learn from our leading authorities that 99 percent of the American people are deficient in these minerals, and that a marked deficiency in any one of the more important minerals actually results in DISEASE. Any upset of the balance, any considerable lack of one or another element, however microscopic the body requirement may be, and we sicken, suffer, and shorten our lives.

Certainly our physical well being is more directly dependent upon the minerals we take in to our system than upon calories or vitamins or upon the precise proportions of starch, protein or carbohydrates we consume.

So it goes, each mineral element playing a definite role in nutrition. A characteristic set of symptoms, just as specific as any vitamin deficiency disease, follows a deficiency in any one of them. It is alarming, therefore, to face the fact that we are starving for these precious health-giving substances.

Sick soils mean sick plants, sick animals, and sick people. Physical, mental and moral fitness depends largely upon an ample supply and a proper proportion of minerals in our foods. Nerve function, nerve stability and nerve cell-building likewise depend upon trace minerals.

Neither does the layman realize that there may be a pronounced difference in both foods and soils - to him one vegetable, one glass of milk, or one egg is about the same as another. Dirt is dirt, too, and he assumes that by adding a little fertilizer to it, a satisfactory vegetable or fruit can be grown.

The truth is that our foods vary enormously in value, and some of them aren't worth eating as food. For example, vegetation grown in one part of the US may assay 1,100 parts per billion of iodine, as against 20 in that grown elsewhere. Processed milk has run anywhere from 362 parts per million of iodine and 127 of iron, down to nothing.

Some of our lands, even in a virgin state, never were well balanced in mineral content, and unhappily for us, we have been systematically robbing the poor soils and the good soils alike of the very substances necessary to health, growth, long life, and resistance to disease. Up to the time I began experimenting, almost nothing had been done to make good the theft. The more I studied nutritional problems and the effects of mineral deficiencies upon disease, the more plainly I saw that here lay the most direct approach to better health, and the more important it became in my mind to find a method of restoring those missing minerals to our foods.

Our soils which are seriously deficient in trace minerals, cannot produce plant life competent to maintain our needs, and with the continuous cropping and shipping away of those trace minerals and concentrates, the condition becomes worse.

One sure way to end the American people's susceptibility to infection is to supply through food, a balanced ration of trace minerals. An organism supplied with a diet adequate to, or preferably in excess of, all mineral requirements may so utilize these elements as to produce immunity from infection quite beyond anything we are able to produce artificially by our present method of immunization. You can't make up the deficiency by using a patent medicine or drug.

Prevention of disease is easier, more practical, and more economical than cure. Disease preys most surely and most viciously on the undernourished and unfit plants, animals and human beings alike, and when the importance of these obscure mineral elements is fully realized, the chemistry of life will have to be rewritten. No man knows his mental or bodily capacity, how well he can feel or how long he can live, for we are all cripples and weaklings.

Appendix B

Resources...

For updated resources and information, please visit www.mindmythsbook.com and click on "Resources".

Perspective/Perception

Spontaneous Evolution: Our Positive Future and a Way to Get There From Here by Bruce Lipton, Ph.D.
Thrive (Movie & DVD) by Foster Gamble: www.thrivemovement.com
The Living Matrix Movie: The New Science of Healing, directed by Greg Becker www.thelivingmatrixmovie.com
Commonwealth by Freddy Silva
Question Your Thinking, Change the World by Byron Katie: www.thework.com
The Spontaneous Healing of Belief by Gregg Braden
The Promise of Energy Psychology: Revolutionary Tools for Dramatic Personal Change by David Feinstein, Donna Eden and Gary Craig
Medical Intuition: Your Awakening to Wholeness by C. Norman Shealy, MD
The Energy Healing Experiments: Science Reveals Our Natural Power to Heal by Gary E. Schwartz, Ph.D.
The Five Agreements by Don Miguel Ruiz

The Power of Now by Eckhart Tolle
You Can Heal Your Life by Louise Hay
The Survivors Club: The Secrets and Science that Could Save Your Life by Ben Sherwood

Epigenetics

The Biology of Belief by Bruce Lipton, Ph.D.
The Genie in Your Genes by Dawson Church, Ph.D.
The Wisdom of Your Cells: How Your Beliefs Control Your Biology (audio CD) by Bruce Lipton, Ph.D.
Epigenetics on PBS.org, A NOVA Program: video.pbs.org/video/1525107473/

Energy Therapies/Psychoenergetic Science

Tapas Acupressure Technique with Tapas Fleming: www.tatlife.com

Emotional Freedom Technique: www.garythink.com, www.emofree.com and www.eftuniverse.com
The EFT Manual by Gary Craig
EFT for Back Pain by Gary Craig (paperback)
Operation: Emotional Freedom (DVD about EFT for PTSD): www.operation-emotionalfreedom.com
Try It On Everything by Nick Ortner (EFT used in a variety of cases)
The Field: The Quest for the Secret Force of the Universe by Lynne McTaggart
Psychoenergetic Science: A Second Copernican-Scale Revolution (DVD of a seminar by Professor William A. Tiller, Ph.D.,
Cymatics www.cymaticsource.com and www.cymatics.org
Reconnective Healing with Dr. Eric Pearl: www.thereconnection.com
Global Coherence Initiative: www.glcoherence.org
Institute of Heart Math: heartmath.org

Environment and Health

Fluoride Action Network: www.flouridealert.org
An Inconvenient Tooth: aninconvenienttooth.org
VacTruth: vactruth.com
National Vaccine Information Center: www.nvic.org
Don't Vaccinate Before You Educate by Mayer Eisenstein, MD, JD, MPH
The Greater Good (DVD): www.greatergoodmovie.com
Seeds of Destruction: The Hidden Agenda of Genetic Manipulation by William F. Engdahl
Scientists Under Attack: Genetic Engineering in the Magnetic Field of Money (DVD) by Bertram Verhaag
The World According to Monsanto (DVD) by Marie-Monique Robin
Why in the World are they Spraying?: www.whyintheworldaretheyspraying.com
Farm Wars: http://farmwars.info
The GMO Trilogy (DVD set) by Jeffery M. Smith
Farmageddon (Online Movie and DVD): farmageddonmovie.com
Food, Inc. (Movie and DVD)
Non-GMO Project: www.nongmoproject.org
Genetic Roulette by Jeffery M. Smith
The Case Against Fluoride by Paul Connett, PhD, James Beck, MD, PhD and James Micklem, D.Phil.
Institute for Responsible Technology (about GMO): www.responsibletechnology.org
Excitotoxins: The Taste that Kills by Russell Blaylock, MD
The Cancer Cure that Worked! Fifty Years of Suppression by Barry Lynes
The Gerson Therapy: The Proven Nutritional Program for Cancer and Other Illnesses by Charlotte Gerson and Morton Walker, DPM
Death by Modern Medicine by Carolyn Dean, MD, ND
Starfield B. *Is US health really the best in the world?*. JAMA. 2000; 284(4):483-4, and it can be downloaded freely on the internet in PDF format.

"Death by Medicine" by Gary Null, PhD, Carolyn Dean MD, ND; Martin Feldman, MD; Debora Rasio, MD; and Dorothy Smith, PhD

Governments and Public Policy

Confessions of an Economic Hit Man by John Perkins
The Creature from Jekyll Island by G. Edward Griffin
Tragedy and Hope by Carroll Quigley
Behind the Green Mask: UN Agenda 21 by Rosa Koire
Controlling the Human Mind by Dr. Nick Begich
The Greatest Hoax by United States Senator James Inhofe
The Deliberate Dumbing Down of America: Revised and Abridged Edition by Charlotte Thomson Iserbyt
Dead Wrong: Straight Facts on the Country's Most Controversial Cover-Ups by Richard Belzer
Assessing the Efficacy and Safety of Medical Technologies Washington, DC, Congress of the United States, Office of Technology Assessment, Publication No. 052003-00593-0. Government Printing Office, Washington, DC, 20402, 1978.)
Healthcare Technology and Its Assessment in Eight Countries February 1995, Government Printing Office stock # 052-003-01402-5 and available online at www.fas.org/ota/reports/9562.pdf

Healing Concepts: Non-Medical

The Hummingbird's Journey to God by Ross Heaven
Iboga: www.ibogahouse.com
Ayahuasca: www.ayahuascaassociation.org

Non-Mainstream News Outlets...

The Drudge Report www.drudgereport.com
Natural News www.naturalnews.com
Russia Today www.rt.com/news
The BBC www.BBC.com/news